Jewish Answers
to
Medical Ethics
Questions

Jewish Answers to Medical Ethics Questions

QUESTIONS AND ANSWERS FROM THE
MEDICAL ETHICS DEPARTMENT
OF THE OFFICE OF THE
CHIEF RABBI OF GREAT BRITAIN

NISSON E. SHULMAN

JASON ARONSON INC.
Northvale, New Jersey
Jerusalem

This book was set in 11 pt. New Baskerville by Hightech Data Inc., of Bangalore, India and printed and bound by Book-mart Press, Inc. of North Bergen, NJ.

10 9 8 7 6 5 4 3 2 1

Library of Congress Cataloging-in-Publication Data

Shulman, Nisson E.
 Jewish answers to medical ethics questions: what people want to
know / by Nisson E. Shulman.
  p. cm.
 "Questions and answers from the Medical Ethics Department of the
 Office of the Chief Rabbi of Great Britain."
 Includes bibliographical references and index.
 ISBN 0-7657-6016-9
 1. Medicine—Religious aspects—Judaism. 2. Medical ethics.
3. Ethics, Jewish. 4. Medical laws and legislation (Jewish law)
I. Office of the Chief Rabbi of Great Britain. Medical Ethics Dept.
II. Title.
R725.57.S58 1998
296.3'642—dc21   98–5337

Printed in the United States of America. Jason Aronson Inc. offers books and cassettes. For information and catalog write to Jason Aronson Inc., 230 Livingston Street, Northvale, NJ 07647-1726, or visit our website: http://www.aronson.com

Contents

Preface

Medical ethics, like other branches of ethical inquiry, does not stand alone. It takes its place within a larger conception of human life. It belongs, in other words, to the great traditions through which humanity has tried to understand its relationship to nature and that which lies beyond nature. As the scope and reach of technology expands, giving us unprecedented power to shape our destiny, so the guidance of those traditions becomes progressively more important in helping us steer a course through ever more fateful choices while remaining faithful to the commitments of our moral and spiritual heritage.

The Jewish tradition contains a remarkable body of ethical reflection. It begins with the Hebrew Bible, perhaps the most influential book in the history of civilization. It continues through the Mishnah and Talmud, the great anthologies of early rabbinic thought. It is further articulated in the literature of the Responsa, through which individual rabbis, after the close of the talmudic era, answered specific questions of Jewish law. Thus for more than three millennia, Jews have reflected on matters of life and death, healing, and the dilemmas it poses, guided at all times by the principles and values set out in our sacred texts.

Those values give Jewish medical ethics its distinctive character, much of it already implicit in the opening chapters of the book of Genesis. Human life, cast as it is in "the image of God," is sacred. Procreation—bringing new life into the world—is the first command with which mankind is charged. Humanity is given the power to "conquer" nature, but at the same time the responsibility "to serve and protect" it. In the powerful rabbinic phrase, man and God are to become "partners in the work of creation."

The task of healing is therefore seen by the Jewish tradition not as an impious attempt to subvert the course of nature or Providence, but as a religious obligation, a way of enhancing life and its dignity. At the same time life is seen as the gift of God. It is not something we own, subject only to our autonomous choices. Rather it is something which has been placed in our safekeeping, and this has implications for Jewish approaches to abortion and euthanasia. The practice of medicine is above all a moral undertaking, and one held in high religious esteem. Indeed some of Judaism's greatest sages—most notably Moses Maimonides—were distinguished physicians. In their writings, medical expertise and reverence for Jewish law interrelate most fully, laying detailed groundwork for a Judaic approach to the complex issues of contemporary medical practice and research.

In recent years, because of the fateful scope of biotechnology, there has been great interest in medical ethics generally, and the Jewish tradition specifically. The work of my predecessor, Lord Jakobovits, played a considerable part in making that tradition widely available to an English-speaking public. Our Office is often consulted on questions of medical ethics, and for many years under both Lord Jakobovits' Chief Rabbinate and my own, answers to those questions were prepared by Rabbi Dr. Nisson Shulman, whose expertise in this field made him eminently suited to the task. He has now assembled those responses, and they form the substance of this book.

The sheer range of this volume makes it an outstanding introduction to Jewish medical ethics as it engages with contemporary dilemmas. Rabbi Shulman is a masterly exponent of the Judaic tradition, and in his hands we see the full power of an ancient tradition to guide us through the complex problems of today. Relevant, articulate, and rich in compelling insights, this is a fine addition to the growing literature on Judaism and medicine, and I am delighted that it will now be available to a wide circle of readers.

—Rabbi Dr. Jonathan Sacks
Chief Rabbi of the United Hebrew
Congregations of the Commonwealth

Foreword

Jewish medical ethics has come of age. The very phrase was unknown until the late 1950s. There existed no literature whatsoever in the vernacular, no textbooks, manuals, or even articles to guide doctors, nurses, medical students, and hospital staff on Jewish insights and laws governing the ethics of their profession. Those in search of Jewish teaching on the subject had to be among the few conversant with the intricacies of rabbinic thinking and writing.

All this has changed dramatically over the past four decades. By now a sizeable collection of comprehensive books, popular and specialized articles, entries in encyclopedias, and even regular periodicals can be assembled in this field. Jewish medical ethics is now an acknowledged discipline of Judaism, alongside long-established subjects like Jewish jurisprudence, Jewish philosophy, and Jewish art.

Spectacular advances in medicine have presented numerous moral problems unthinkable in the past and have provoked fierce public and professional debate. Judaism has much to say about these problems, and its insights are vital to true moral solutions based on the immensely rich Jewish heritage in the field of medicine and Jewish law.

There is an ever-growing number of deeply committed Jews entering the medical profession. They rely on an authentic presentation of their own tradition for solutions to the many ethical problems they are bound to encounter. They also frequently bring a rich background of our tradition with them and contribute much to the insights we perceive and the solutions we seek.

Of all the sciences, it is pre-eminently medicine that enjoys a natural kinship with Judaism historically and intellectually. For many centuries, rabbis and physicians, often merging their professions into one, were intimate partners in a common effort for the betterment of life. This partnership has been enhanced through the Medical Ethics Centre at Jews' College.

I am very grateful to Rabbi Dr. Nisson Shulman for his work in medical ethics while serving on my Rabbinic Cabinet when I was Chief Rabbi, work he continued under the encouragement and leadership of my successor, Rabbi Jonathan Sacks. He had undertaken the monumental task of editing the first two years of Jews' College Medical Ethics seminars and preparing selections of the proceedings for publication. He has now undertaken to edit and publish selected responses that came from the Chief Rabbi's office where he was entrusted with the task of responding to Medical Ethics inquiries from many parts of the world.

—Lord Immanuel Jakobovits, Chief Rabbi Emeritus and Patron of the Centre for Medical Ethics, Jews' College, London

Introduction

In 1988 Lord Immanuel Jakobovits, then the Chief Rabbi of the British Commonwealth, appointed me to his Rabbinic Cabinet to be in charge of the section on Medical Ethics. I helped to answer some of the many questions in this field that came to him. When Dr. Jonathan Sacks became Chief Rabbi he reconfirmed this appointment and expanded the scope of the work so that I became spokesman for Medical Ethics in his cabinet. I was thus involved with these questions for more than six years.

I checked all controversial responses with the Chief Rabbi, or, by his instruction, with his Rabbinical Court, the Beth Din of London. I often checked with experts overseas as well. In this I was greatly aided by having recognized experts available, such as Lord Jakobovits, Dayan Ehrentreu, Dayan Berger, Rabbi Moshe Dovid Tendler, and sources written in a number of excellent modern collections, such as those by Dr. Fred Rosner, Rabbi J. David Bleich, Dr. Abraham Abraham, Dr. Mordecai Halperin, and others. Where a discussion of original sources is helpful, I cite them, but as briefly as possible, for the book is intended for the layman seeking to learn Judaism's view on issues of concern to doctors and the general public.

These replies are not *pesak halakhah*. The vast majority of the questions are not *sheelot*, questions of Jewish law in the true sense of the word. *Sheelot* deal with specific problems and require answers that determine a course of action. These are rather inquiries about Judaism's point of view in general matters that relate to burning issues of the times and come from people in all walks of life, laymen and professionals, groups, and even government agencies. Some were socially or politically sensitive.

For example: the Chief Rabbi of the Sephardic Community of Tel Aviv had, according to newspaper reports, outlawed wearing fur and the fur trade because of unwarranted cruelty to animals. LYNX, the organization seeking to ban the fur trade, asked Chief Rabbi Sacks to make a statement supporting this and to forbid Jews in Britain to wear fur. It was a delicate issue. The answer was given to the Chief Rabbi for approval and revision before being sent.[1] Another example: the Ministry of Agriculture, Food, and Fisheries (MAFF) wanted to know the Jewish view of genetically modified food in the food chain. Again, after the reply was prepared, it was given to members of the Beth Din as well as the Chief Rabbi for approval.[2] In answering these questions I referred to the vast literature that has grown in this area. Often I would include reprints of articles and even, with permission, chapters of books.

I was also called upon to present the halakhic view on medical issues to the wider community through lectures and articles and by organizing conferences and other special events. On occasion, there was the opportunity to participate with special-interest groups such as the anti-euthanasia lobby and the Human Values in Health Care Discussion Group, a symposium

1. See infra, p. 215.
2. See infra, p. 14.

of ethicists and physicians formed to analyze how medicine could degenerate as it did under the Nazi regime. They also sought to advocate for public policy and action that would help prevent such degeneration from ever happening again.

In 1994 I left the United Kingdom to become part of the administration of the Rabbi Isaac Elchanan Theological Seminary affiliated with Yeshiva University in New York. This compilation is selected from the Medical Ethics responsa I wrote during my six and a half "British" years.

Judaism has a great contribution to make to the field of medical ethics. In the words of the *Compendium on [Jewish] Medical Ethics:*

> Jewish ethics represents the accumulated wisdom and intellectual labor of millennia, stretching from the Bible and the Talmud, through the codes of Jewish Law, to the most recent and contemporary rabbinic essays and responsa. . . . The wisdom distilled from 3500 years of study and governance of human affairs, which comprises a large part of the Jewish Code of Law, yields specific directives for moral behavior in all of the great ethical dilemmas facing medicine and society today.[3]

Judaism has important views on organ transplants, genetic engineering, abortion, new birth techniques, surrogate parenthood, contemporary psychiatric practices, allocation of scarce resources, the moment of death, the care of the critically ill, and so on. Judaism's views on understanding and resolving modern issues of medical ethics are becoming better known. The above-mentioned *Compendium on Medical Ethics*, published by the Federation of Jewish Philanthropies Medical Ethics Commission and now in its sixth revision, is used in many major hospitals throughout the United States and in

---

3. David Feldman and Dr. Fred Rosner (ed), *Compendium on Medical Ethics*, (Federation of Jewish Philanthropies of New York, 1986), Sixth Edition, pp. 5, 11.

many parts of the world. The Mount Sinai Medical Center has conducted an annual conference on Jewish Medical Ethics for all health-care specialists in the New York area and has devoted the fiftieth-anniversary issue (1984) of its *Journal of Medicine* entirely to reprinting papers that highlighted the previous decade of this conference. A major conference on Jewish Medical Ethics takes place annually in San Francisco. As far off as Australia, the Fellowship of Jewish Doctors of New South Wales and its counterpart in Victoria are making contributions to the field. A growing literature dealing with the Jewish point of view on medical ethical issues is emerging, especially in Israel and in America.

Even so, the number of those familiar with the medical ethical views of Judaism is still relatively small, in fact a tiny minority of those involved in health care, and certainly of the population at large. This makes it increasingly important to bring the contribution Judaism can offer to the attention of everyone who can benefit by it.

Many of the issues discussed in this book are also found in the vast literature developed and developing on this subject. The purpose of this volume is to organize and collect answers to questions most frequently asked. The answers are organized according to the queries that came to my attention, and areas about which I did not receive questions are not included. On the other hand, many of the questions dealt with have been asked repeatedly and are therefore to be considered very much on today's agenda.

I am grateful to Rabbi Moshe Dovid Tendler for being constantly available for consultation, for encouraging me to work on this project, and for his valuable comments on the final manuscript, and to Dr. Fred Rosner for his help in reading the manuscript and offering his own very valuable suggestions.

I am also grateful to Dr. Norman Lamm, President of Yeshiva University, for his inspiration, friendship, and encouragement.

—Nisson E. Shulman

1

The Obligation to Heal

Question: A member of the Royal College of Physicians, Edinburgh, asked for chapter and verse of Biblical passages where Judaism discusses a doctor's duty to heal. "A physician," he said, "as a scientist, believes it is his mandate to heal. But yours is a religion. Why do you not hold with those faiths that declare that healing is wholly in God's hands?"

Answer: The following reply is based on three verses as interpreted by the Rabbis. Rabbi Moshe Dovid Tendler points out that the verses are actually a progression, and must be understood as follows:[1]

The first source is Exodus 21:19. "You shall surely heal," which is the commandment and permission for man to intervene in the healing process. Were it not for such a Biblical imperative, it would be an act of audacity on the part of a

---

1. Moshe D. Tendler, *First Sydney Conference of Jewish Bioethics*, ed. Nisson E. Shulman, (August 1987), pp. 31ff.

human being to intervene: "if God made people sick, how dare you try to make them well?" Some groups do accept that notion as an article of their faith and hence have rejected medical ministrations in favor of a theological approach to the cure of disease.

The second verse is Deuteronomy 22:2, referring to a lost object, where God commands: "Return [it] to him—you shall not hide your eyes [from it]." You have a duty to return lost objects, from which the Rabbis infer that if you must return his lost object, how much more must you return his lost health? Hence is derived the imperative commanding us to return a person's lost health. While the first verse might be thought to refer only to physicians who have the skill to heal, the verse about lost property indicates that everyone who can give some kind of help must do so, a kind of "Good Samaritan" law.

The third verse is Leviticus 19:17. It reads: "Do not stand idly by when your neighbor's blood is flowing." This implies an additional commitment. You are required to take a modicum of risk in order to help someone in trouble. Not only are you required to throw a life ring to someone who is drowning, you are also required, when necessary, to jump in after him, provided the risk to your own life is small. Furthermore, you are required to expend funds in order to save him.

On the basis of these verses, Rabbi J. David Bleich contrasts the legal system of our country, in which the relationship between a physician and his patient is purely contractual, so that a doctor has the absolute legal right to refuse to treat a patient who is not yet under his care,[2] and in fact may not, except in an emergency, treat patients without their consent[3]—with Jewish law, according to which we have a respon-

---

2. J. David Bleich, *Judaism and Healing*, Ktav Publishing Co, (New York 1981), p. 11.

3. Ibid., p. 18–20.

sibility to heal the patient beyond that of legal contract.[4]

Rabbi Bleich cites later sages who add additional sources to the requirement to heal. Thus Nahmanides states that the obligation to heal is inherent in the commandment "And you shall love your neighbor as yourself" (Leviticus 19:18).[5] In his Bible commentary on Leviticus 25:36 he adds the source "And your brother shall live with you" as constituting a general obligation to preserve the life of one's fellow. The Talmud (*Yoma* 85b) renders this passage as meaning "And he shall live through them [the commandments] but he shall not die by [means of] them," and, accordingly, this verse is understood to establish the principle that *mitzvot* are suspended in the face of life-threatening dangers.[6]

But now a new question arises. May a physician refuse someone treatment, for instance an AIDS victim, because of fear of infection? Here the personal danger is in conflict with the commandment to heal. *Venishmartem meod lenafshosechem*,[7] "Guard your own selves from harm," is also a Torah commandment just as is the duty to heal. Which takes precedence? Of course, a doctor who is sensitive to *halakhah* will take all proper precautions and will not refuse such a patient. But what about a patient whose social conduct puts him at special risk of contracting that disease? Suppose the doctor knows the patient is a drug addict who might have been using contaminated needles. Can the doctor insist that, if he is

---

4. Hizkiyahu Avraham Broide, "Hovat Harofe Lahole . . ." Assia 51–52, Vol. 13, Iyar 5752 for a discussion of whether a doctor must force healing on a patient over his objection.

5. Bleich, Contemporary Halakhic Problems, Vol. II, (Ktav Publishing Co. and Yeshiva University Press, New York 1983), p. 4ff.

6. Ibid., p. 55.

7. Deut. 4:15. Although the primary meaning is to guard against idolatry, the rabbis have also taken this to mean that a person must guard his health as well as his soul. Maimonides, in Mishneh Torah, "*Hilchot Deot*" 4:1, stresses that a sound body is necessary in order to serve the Almighty properly.

to risk his own life to care for that patient, the least that patient can be expected to do is to take a blood test to indicate
to that doctor whether he must take those extra precautions
in treating that particular patient? Suppose the doctor insists
that he wants to be reassured, and taking a blood test is a
small enough assurance for him to require. There are halakhic
opinions that free the doctor from the requirement to care
for that patient unless the patient does as the doctor requests.[8]
After all, though you are commanded to help your neighbor
who is struggling under an unmanageable burden such as
loading a pack onto an animal, you are not required to help
if he should stand idly by, fold his hands, and say, "You are
commanded to help, so you do it all."[9] In similar fashion the
doctor can require of an at-risk patient some measure of co-
operation in return for his undertaking the risk of treating
him.

8. Immanuel Jakobovits, in a private conversation with me.
9. Talmud Babli, *Baba Metzia*, 32a.

2

Genetic Issues

Genetics

Question (From Dr. Malcolm Eames, then Head of Research and Information, British Union for the Abolition of Vivisection, now Research Fellow, SPRU):

I noticed your letter in the *Journal of Chemistry and Industry* (June 21, 1993) in response to Dr. Linzey's essay on Christianity and animal patenting. As you may be aware, The British Union for the Abolition of Vivisection, together with Compassion in World Farming, have lodged formal opposition to the granting of a European patent on the "Harvard Oncomouse."

I note that your letter stated that you did not see any ethical difference between the genetic modification of animals and plants by selective breeding and by the use of genetic engineering techniques, provided that there were "adequate guarantees against violation of human safety and prevention of unnecessary cruelty to animals." I would be interested to learn whether you consider that the development of animal genetic engineering raises any particular ethical questions from a Jewish perspective over and above those relating to animal pat-

11

enting. For example, would you consider that the insertion of human genetic material into another species—such as in the case of the group of Cambridge scientists who are attempting to produce "humanized" trans-genic pigs for use as organ donors—raises any particular ethical questions or concerns. Thank you for your assistance with this matter.

Another question on the same subject adds the following comment: " 'In the beginning,' we are told, 'God created heaven and earth and every living creature that moveth on the waters and that creepeth upon the earth' (Genesis 1), but not according to the European Patent Office. Living creatures can now be classed as 'inventions' designed by humans."

Answer: Additional questions on this subject have been received and will be discussed in greater detail in the section to follow. My letter, printed in the issue of the *Journal of Chemistry and Industry* to which Mr. Eames refers, answers the query about the Oncomouse, a mouse genetically engineered to be susceptible to human forms of cancer, bred to be used in cancer research. Following is the text of that letter:

> In a recent essay Dr. Linzey explained why Christianity opposes modifications of nature for therapy as represented by the "Oncomouse." Judaism's view is quite different.
>
> Judaism agrees that there is a need to protect the species and the ecology of the world. At the same time another, seemingly contradictory, value requires man to use nature and advance with science. He is required to fill the natural world and subdue it for his needs—to "hold dominion over the fish of the sea and the birds of the air and every living thing crawling on the earth" (Gen. 1:28). He is entitled to exploit animals in his service and for his health, provided they are protected from all avoidable suffering. The delicate balance struck by these two seemingly contradictory imperatives has

been addressed by Judaism for thousands of years. Several principles emerge from this age-old discussion.

1. Man is given a task to use nature for his benefit and a responsibility to nurture and protect it. For the world was purposely created with imperfections so that man can join with Almighty God in perfecting this world, thus becoming a partner with God in creation.

2. Man has a religious duty to heal. Saving life takes precedence over almost all Biblical and Rabbinic commandments and disciplines. Many life-saving and life-prolonging products can be manufactured through genetic engineering.

3. We see no ethical difference between genetic modification of animals and plants by selective breeding and doing so in the laboratory with new scientific techniques, provided that there are adequate and failsafe guarantees against violation of human safety and prevention of unnecessary cruelty to animals.

4. There is no objection to new products such as the "Oncomouse" for use in laboratory experiments in order to cure illness, since man is given dominion over this world which is created for his use.

5. The use of this world must be for benign purposes. Unnecessary pain must be avoided. Judaism has very strict requirements to prevent undue pain and avoid all cruelty to animals.

6. May the "Oncomouse" be patented and owned? Judaism limits ownership of life forms. It forbids such ownership entirely in human life, so that one person cannot be enslaved to serve another and one life cannot be sacrificed for another. Judaism does permit ownership of animals and other forms of life. But it would severely limit, and even forbid, ownership of "types" of life, such as a species. The "Oncomouse" therefore may not be "owned."

Actually, man owns nothing in this world. "The earth is the Lord's and the fullness thereof"[1] is understood by Jewish tradition to mean that everything in this world belongs to God and nothing to man. Man holds it in trust for humankind's benefit and for the protection of this world. Patenting as a reward for human ingenuity can apply to genetic manipulations and permutations. But it should not lead to ownership of a form or type of life, for this would be contrary to the spirit of the Lord's ownership of the world and everything in it.

Mr. Eames' question obviously goes beyond the issue of patenting a "life form," which would be objectionable. He is actually asking about the entire area of genetic modification of plants and animals, and particularly in regard to food production. That question is answered in the following section.

Questions: A much more elaborate query came from Tim Davis, Secretary to the Ministry of Agriculture, Food, and Fisheries Study Group on Genetic Modification Programs and Food Use. The Nuffield Foundation has a task force engaged in similar research, and their Secretary, Mr. David Shapiro, asked similar questions. I later testified before the MAFF Study Group at their request. Following is a summary of their questions:

1. May the results of genetically modified foods be used in the food chain?
2. Do human genes or genetic material retain "humanity" upon transfer to another organism?
3. May we eat such genetically modified organisms?
4. If genes or genetic material from animals forbidden to Jews are transferred to modify permitted animals, does this render the animals forbidden?

---

1. Psalms 24:1.

5. Does modification of plant growth by genetic material from animal sources render the plant "non-vegetarian"?

6. May animals be fed with genetically modified material, especially if modified with human genes?

7. What form of control should be instituted for this kind of genetic modification of foods to be used in the food chain?

8. What about cruelty to animals?

9. Does Judaism have anything to say about ownership of such new material, patenting of life forms, for instance?

10. Would the rabbis require labelling the products as having been genetically modified?

Answer: The problem of modification of species is not new. We are biblically required to "preserve the world and to tend it." (Genesis 2:15) We are also required to use it for our benefit. The delicate balance struck by these two seemingly contradictory imperatives has been addressed by Judaism for thousands of years.

We therefore welcome the great concern now shown by government, scientific groups, and the public to preserve the ecology and protect the world we live in, as well as humanity. Although genetic engineering is not technically the same as cross-breeding of species, nevertheless the spirit of the Biblical law requires that adequate safeguards be set in place so that this technique may be used in the service of human beings rather than in upsetting, harming, and even ultimately destroying the natural world. It is gratifying that your inquiry is in the spirit of Biblical imperative and that it seeks, as one of its major concerns, to protect human beings and their environment, thus facing a problem that Judaism perceives to be as old as humanity itself.

Following are some principles Judaism maintains, along with answers to your questions based on those principles.

Man is given a task on earth to use nature for his benefit, and, as a steward of the Almighty, is responsible for nurturing and protecting it. For the world was purposely created imperfect so that man can join with Almighty God in perfecting it. In so doing, he becomes "a partner with God in creation." Man must advance with the advance of science. He builds bridges, conquers floods, develops new methods of irrigation, manufacture, and creative art. He crosses oceans and creates machines that conquer the air and ultimately the far reaches of space. In all this he conquers, uses, and even changes the natural world. And among his most important mandates is to heal the sick. For Judaism does not believe that naturalness is necessarily a virtue.

> There are other faiths and groups that have made a virtue of the natural, the unnatural being unclean or unholy. To Judaism, the artificial may well be the greatest human contribution, sanctioned by God and welcomed by man. The artificial kidney, the artificial heart, artificial insemination, and artificial respiration are, at the same time, our duty and our obligation as well as our right and privilege. They may very well involve the greatest *mitzvot*, the greatest "good deeds" of a physician.[2]

Man has a religious duty to heal. Saving life takes precedence over almost all of the commandments and disciplines of the Torah, both Biblical and Rabbinic. Many life-saving and life-prolonging products can be manufactured through genetic engineering. This opens a marvelous new window to the future, enabling us to fulfill still more nobly our responsibility towards the Creator, towards this world, towards saving and prolonging human life.[3]

In actual fact, laboratory production of genetically modified organisms may be even more acceptable than selective

---

2. Moshe D. Tendler, "Rabbinic Comment: Transplantation Surgery," *The Mount Sinai Journal of Medicine*, Vol. 51, No. 1, (New York January-February 1984), p. 54.
3. *Compendium of Medical Ethics*, pp. 62–63.

breeding and cross-breeding, since, where Judaism forbids the actual process of cross-breeding, it still permits the resulting product. It is likely that, if done genetically, even the process itself would be permitted.

The genetic material is considered part of the host. It is not regarded as a part of the donor organism at all. In the same way gonad transplants become part of the host, even if they bear genetic resemblance (sperm, for instance) to the donor.[4] A permitted food would therefore not become forbidden simply because of gene modification. Cloven hooves and cud chewing are both necessary to render an animal kosher. Genetic modifications will not render an animal that is other-

---

4. Feldman and Rosner, 1986, op. cit., pp. 70–71. There is Rabbinic discussion and disagreement regarding host mothers by whose nurture the baby is brought to term, and on the other hand the biological mother—the donor of the egg—whose nature determines the genetic composition of the offspring. Rabbi M. Feinstein suggests that, though the majority opinion holds the host mother to be the parent, one must also take into account the maternal relationship of the biological mother. Jewish law would then accept both relationships, ruling strictly in each case. For instance; sexual relations with a sibling from either mother would be considered possible incest. While in cases of transplant surgery the body part belongs to the host, and here too the host mother would be considered the parent, nevertheless the special nature of ovarian transplant makes it appropriate *also* to consider the possibility of a biological relationship with the donor. For, as Rosner (1986) points out, there may be a difference between an ovarian transplant and testicular transplant, for the sperm are to be produced in the future. The ovary, however, already contains the primordial egg cells at the time of the transplant. Though the gamete maintains its own individuality and retains the genetic code of the donor without reflecting the genetic code of the recipient, the fact remains that the sperm is manufactured by the host, while the eggs were already present at the time of transplant. It would therefore be consistent to say that even gonad transplants become part of the host.

wise kosher into a non-kosher animal unless it modifies those two requirements (rendering the cloven hoof into a single hoof or eliminating cud chewing). The only other way a genetic variation can render a kosher animal non-kosher is by threatening the life of the host animal, since any animal that would not otherwise have survived a minimum of twelve months is considered not kosher.[5] Furthermore, Judaism does not regard genes as "food," so that the introduction of a gene or genetic material from non-kosher animals would not render the recipient non-kosher.

The human body is a trust given to us, making us its guardians. It does not belong to us but to God who gave it. We cannot wilfully harm it or destroy it. Suicide is therefore forbidden. We may not even make a scratch on our bodies except for therapeutic reasons, for we would be harming the body God gave us in trust. We may therefore eat otherwise kosher genetically modified plants and animals only if they are safe to eat, and must institute adequate safeguards to prevent harmful effects of the products of genetic modification. Safeguards have been instituted in gene therapy. Dr. Fred Rosner, in an article in the *New York State Journal of Medicine* out-

---

5. There are actually eighteen listed pathologies or anomolies, perforations, or wounds that render an animal *treifa*, "torn," and therefore not kosher to eat (Talmud, Hulin, 42a). Depending on the classification style, the number can be reduced to eight more general types (Shulchan Aruch Yore Deah, "*Hilchot Treifot*," 29:1), or seventy more specific types (Maimonides, "Hilchot Shechita," 10:9). They are all derived from an oral tradition that derives from Mount Sinai. For that reason we do not add to these *treifot* nor subtract from their number. While animals that are free of these eighteen wounds or sicknesses are not, by definition, considered *treifa*, as Maimonides clearly states (10:12, 13), nevertheless the spirit of Jewish law can be said to extend the prohibition, making any sick animal that cannot survive a twelvemonth into a questionable state of *treifa* at least by rabbinic decree, and therefore one that should not be eaten.

lines the benefits and hazards of genetic engineering and indicates some safeguards that enable that science to proceed.[6] Similar safeguards should be instituted to protect foods and to insure that there are no harmful side effects. The food and drug acts of various countries work effectively.

Since Jewish law considers the host's character as dominant, there would be no prohibition against eating plants genetically modified with animal or human genes. They would still be considered vegetarian.

If the food is permitted as kosher, modified and non-modified strains would be equally kosher, provided adequate safeguards had been instituted to prevent harmful effects from ensuing. It would also be advisable to embark on a program of public education to teach that there is no difference between the product genetically modified in the laboratory and the product genetically modified by selective breeding.

Jewish law would make no objection to new products such as the "Oncomouse" for use in laboratory experiments in order to cure illness, since Man is given dominion over this world that is created for his use. There are, of course, reservations. One is that the use of this world must be for benign purposes. Another is that the new products must be developed for serious reasons, such as for therapy, and not for frivolous reasons.[7] This requirement is met by the "Oncomouse," since its creation and use are for cancer cure.

Another reservation is that unnecessary cruelty must be avoided. Judaism has very strict requirements for preventing undue pain and avoiding all cruelty to animals. It opposes hunting and trapping for pleasure, but allows animal use for commercial as well as therapeutic purposes, provided everything possible be done to eliminate or minimize the

---

6. Fred Rosner, "Recombinant DNA...", *NY State Journal of Medicine* 1979, Vol. 79 No. 9, pp. 1439–44.
7. See *Time* magazine, May 30, 1994, for a description of some of the frivolous uses to which genetic engineering has been put.

animals' pain.[8]

Another issue raised by the "Oncomouse" is patenting and ownership. Judaism limits ownership of life forms. It forbids such ownership entirely in human life, so that one person cannot be enslaved to serve another, and one life cannot be sacrificed for another. For that reason donations of life-saving organs that would cause death by removal can be harvested only after the moment of death. Judaism does permit the ownership of animals and other forms of life. And it would also condone "use" patents that allow scientists to benefit from their ingenuity. A fine line must be drawn between a "use" patent and one that would attribute "ownership" to a type or form of life. Ownership of a particular species would fall under the latter category.

In the same way Judaism would limit the ownership of tissue modified for therapeutic purposes, since the body is not ours but given to us in stewardship. Lord Jakobovits is of the opinion that Judaism might consider the owner as not having property rights in the tissue at all, but only stewardship obligations. This would also apply to genetically modified material.[9]

Dayan Berger, a past senior Rabbinical Court Judge on the London Rabbinical Court (Beth Din), disagrees and holds that just as there are stewardship obligations in the case of tissue, there are stewardship rights as well, and that the rights of quasi-ownership do apply.[10]

---

8. See Rosner, "Animal Experimentation," *Modern Medicine and Jewish Ethics* (1986), pp. 321–337; C. Roth, "Cruelty to Animals," in *Encyclopaedia Judaica* (1972), vol. 3, cols. 5–7; I. Jakobovits, "The Medical Treatment of Animals in Jewish Law," *Journal of Jewish Studies* 7 (1956): 207–220; J. David Bleich, *Judaism and Healing* (New York: Ktav, 1981), pp. 123–125.
9. Lord Immanuel Jakobovits, *personal communication*.
10. Dayan Isaac Berger, *personal communication*.

Question: I am a third-year undergraduate studying Biological Sciences at the University of Warwick. I have recently undertaken a project to investigate social attitudes to gene therapy. I would like to hear about the social attitude of your community on two points:

1. Is there an ethical violation in the replacement of defective genes with healthy substitutes in non-reproductive tissue (*e.g.*, lung or liver cells)?
2. Does Judaism allow us to manipulate genetic material to select desirable traits in our offspring?

Answer: We recognize the dangers inherent in genetic manipulation and genetic engineering. The benefits are so great that we are willing to face the dangers inherent in this new science, provided we protect ourselves with all possible safeguards. We encourage use of the knowledge and skills to cure disease. Selecting "desirable" traits in order to manufacture more nearly perfect humans, however, is forbidden. Many have written on the subject.[11]

Following is an excerpt from a joint statement about genetic engineering I drafted together with Dr. Lionel Kopelowitz, then Chairman of the British Board of Jewish Deputies:[12]

---

11. See especially Fred Rosner's *Modern Medicine and Jewish Ethics* (1979), pp 176ff. There is a section in the Compendium on [Jewish] Medical Ethics entitled "Medical Genetics", and an excellent article (also by Rosner) in *The New York State Journal of Medicine* entitled "Recombinant DNA, Cloning, Genetic Engineering and Judaism." There are also two chapters by Fred Rosner and Azriel Rosenfeld, in *Jewish Bioethics* (Sanhedrin Press, New York and London, 1979), ed. Fred Rosner and J. David Bleich, pp. 401ff.
12. Not published.

The issues involved in "genetic engineering" (recombinant DNA research) involve important concerns for Judaism, and indeed for all mankind.

Because of these new techniques which enable scientists to transfer genes to totally unrelated hosts and by means of a vector—usually a virus—to transfer DNA material into the animal, plant, or bacterial cell of choice, medical science now has the capacity to rearrange the genetic heritage of thousands of years.

The advantages and disadvantages to society are clearly summarised in an article by Dr. Fred Rosner, "Recombinant DNA, Cloning, Genetic Engineering and Judaism."[13] The article gives a picture of great benefit and equally great potential harm, depending on how this science develops and how it is used.

More dangerous still is the potential of nuclear transplants, or "cloning." If an egg's nucleus is replaced by another from any cell in a human body, the genetic code of that nucleus, which had been only half complete, waiting for the other half through fertilization, has now a complete set of chromosomes and proceeds to reproduce on the basis of the new and complete genetic code with which it has been furnished. It can come to term, virtually without conception, using only a male or female seed, not both. It is birth from one parent only. Horrifying consequences can ensue, and some of them are listed in Dr. Rosner's article. The values of Judaism that must guide and limit such research and manipulation have been stated in Lord Jakobovits' submission to the Warnock Commission,[14] as well as in his address to the House of Lords.[15]

---

13. *Supra*, p. 19, n. 6.
14. I. Jakobovits, *Human Fertilisation and Embryology—A Jewish View* "Submissions to the Warnock Committee of Inquiry and The Department of Health and Social Security," (Office of the Chief Rabbi, London, 184), 22 pages.
15. I. Jakobovits, "Embryology Bill," *House of Lords Official Report*, (Parliamentary Debates, Hansard, London, March 6, 1990), pp. 1059ff.

a. Since human life is of infinite value, it cannot be tampered with to manipulate or change its nature. "Man makes many coins from one stamp," says the Mishnah, "and each is exactly like the other. But God makes many humans from the same person and each is different. Each is a unique personality. Therefore let each individual consider that it is as if the whole world was created for him."[16]

b. Cloning, and other kinds of genetic manipulation, treats man like a tool. It is predicated on the human being as a usable, changeable commodity. To Judaism, that is abhorrent. No human may be in another's service. Nor may he be used to serve nature. The wonders of nature were created for man's benefit, and not the other way around.

c. Precisely because human life is of infinite importance, there is a place for genetic science as a means of therapy. Genetic changes may be undertaken to eliminate dread diseases. Manipulation is forbidden; therapy is permitted and encouraged.

It should be added that there is a true and valid fear of where genetic engineering and fertility management can lead. We are concerned with the future, and with how to limit science and assure its being used only for good. The fear is that our society can begin to resemble a "Brave New World," with a new cast of characters, people like Steptoe and Edwards—pioneers in genetic engineering—instead of *Brave New World*'s character, "The Director of Hatcheries."

In his 1974 article, Edwards never mentions the husband's sperm but speaks only of "semen donors." He questions whether donors are legally liable for "wrongful life" should the child come out of the womb damaged. He is not talking about solving the problem of a couple who want a child, but of

---

16. Talmud, Sanhedrin 37a.

solving the problem of a society that wants superior children.

Of greater ethical concern is Edwards' statement that his work opens up the possibility of further work on human embryos in the laboratory, the possibility of cloning them, because in the early stages of cell division each cell has total potency.

> You can divide into quadruplets, or quintuplets, or hundreds, or thousands of identicals. True cloning could go on, . . . by letting the egg fertilize on two good contributors, egg and sperm, separated at the eight cell stage. I could now have eight identical people who can be trained to do the work that I want to train them to do. I could prevent the imbalance of the sexes by recording the sex of newborn children and adjusting the choice open to the parents.[17]

We suddenly have the master of the hatcheries, the president of the organization, declaring that if you want me to help you, you'll have to settle for a girl because my previous customer took a boy and I have to keep a balance. This was a plan long before the first successful child was conceived in vitro, and before the potential of the field of genetic engineering was truly understood.[18]

These are real fears. But it is not sufficient, says Judaism, to halt the application of our knowledge to therapy and the elimination of dread diseases. Judaism declares that man is basically good, and he must be guided, helped, and encouraged to express his stewardship of this world according to the spirit of Godliness planted in him. He is wise and good enough, says Judaism, to be trusted to institute the safeguards

---

17. Steptoe, PC, Edwards RG. "Re-implantation of a Human Embryo With Subsequent Tubal Pregnancy", *Lancet*, 1976; 1:880.
18. Rabbinic Response by Dr. Moshe D. Tendler in the Fiftieth Anniversary Issue of the *Mount Sinai Journal of Medicine*, (January-February, 1984), Vol. 51 No. 1, p. 11.

that will insure the greatest possible benefit with the least possible risk.

The Talmud teaches that there are three partners in man, "the Holy One blessed be He, the father, and the mother. . . ."[19] Man must therefore never be a laboratory product. He is created in the image of his Creator. But he must also be generated and reared by identifiable, human parents, forming a family, who care for and nurture their offspring with love and compassion.[20]

The key point in this discussion is this: if cloning or manipulation of genes is done to "improve" the genome, you put a price tag on individuals. You change individual traits to conform to preconceived values. This is wrong and forbidden by Judaism. On the other hand, you can manipulate genes to "correct" defects in order to provide therapy and to cure disease. This is encouraged by Judaism.

I hope this has helped clarify the Jewish stand in the spirit of the explanations and guidance, as well as the decisions of Jewish law issued by the Emeritus Chief Rabbi, Lord Jakobovits, and the London Beth Din.

19. Talmud, Kiddushin 30b.
20. See Immanuel Jakobovits *Human Fertilization* . . . , and Fred Rosner, Recombinant DNA. . . . *NY State Journal of Medicine* (1979), Vol. 79 No. 9, pp. 1439–1444.

Tinneius Rufus and
Rabbi Akiva

I summarized the material about genetic modifications in a short article in *Le'ela*,[21] including some additional material not found in the above discussion, noting a debate between Tinneius Rufus and Rabbi Akiva that appears in several places in the Talmud and Midrash. These are not the only issues between Tinneius Rufus and Rabbi Akiva, for in several places we find the tyrant questioning him about other matters such as the Jewish calendar, especially the Sabbath and the need for it.[22] The debate about creation is particularly significant because it characterizes the divergent *weltanschauung* of the pagan and the Jewish worlds.

Judaism's approach to man's intervention in nature in order to create a better world can be illustrated by a remarkable discussion recorded in the Talmud which took place in the second century of our era between Tinneius Rufus, the Roman tyrant, and Rabbi Akiva. The tyrant asked three questions

---

21. *Le'ela*, published by Jews' College, London, (September 1994), pp. 20–22.
22. Talmud, Sanhedrin, 65b and Midrash Genesis Rabbah 11.

found in various parts of the Talmud. They all express one idea, one great difference between the pagan and the Jewish approach to man and the world; The tyrant asked, "If God wanted man circumcised, why didn't he create him so?"[23] To which the rabbi answered that God created man with a symbolic imperfection in order that man should join with the Almighty in perfecting himself. In this way man becomes a partner with God in creation. The tyrant continued, "If God loves the poor, why doesn't He feed them?"[24] To which the rabbi responded that this is because God wants us to join with him in perfecting society and so become a partner with God in creation. The tyrant continued, "Which are better, the works of God or the works of man?" The rabbi answered, "The works of man." "Look at the stars in heaven!" exclaimed the tyrant. The rabbi answered, "Look at the wheat; this is the work of God. Look at the bread; this is the work of man." Because real perfection is achieved when man joins his labor with God's work and in this way becomes a partner with God in creation.[25]

To the tyrant the status quo was perfect. There is sickness and death, there are slaves and masters; everything natural is good, the unnatural is not. To the rabbi the natural is only half of creation. The perfection of creation lies in the part man is required to complete. God challenges man to join with Him and complete His work in healing sickness and developing his own potential, in caring for society, and in developing nature's resources, provided he guards this world, tends it, and preserves it, because he is to be a partner with God in the world's creation, not in its destruction.

Note that the tyrant's questions were in three areas: the human body, human society, and the world of nature. In each

---

23. Midrash Tanhuma Leviticus, Tazria 5.
24. Talmud, Baba Batra, 10a.
25. Midrash Tanhuma, loc. cit.

of these areas Tinneius Rufus stated that the highest perfection is to be found in the status quo. To the Jew, the highest perfection is in the creative partnership between God who gives the material of this world and man who is commanded to perfect it.

Biotechnology and Industry

Question: Can you comment on the dangers of biotechnology, especially as it pertains to fields beyond medicine, such as industry?

Answer: Biotechnology is the science of the twenty-first century. According to Michael Crichton, the author of *Jurassic Park*,[26] it promises "the greatest revolution in human history." In his introduction Crichton points out the difference between today's scientific breakthroughs and those of times gone by. He claims that the biotechnological research is broad-based: "America entered the atomic age through the work of a single research institution, at Los Alamos. It entered the computer age through the efforts of about a dozen companies. But biotechnology research is now carried out in more than two thousand laboratories in America alone. Five hundred corporations spend five billion dollars a year on this tech-

---

26. Michael Crichton, *Jurassic Park*, (Random House, New York, 1990), Introduction.

nology" (p. ix). He also notes that the research can be thoughtless, frivolous, and chiefly done for profit. And, finally, he states that while in the past scientists were aloof from commerce, today "there are very few molecular biologists and very few research institutions without commercial affiliations."

Michael Crichton's analysis gives cause for alarm. What is the real situation?

Not long ago I had a chance to deliver an address to a Conference on Bioethics organized by the Chemical Industries Association. I was able to listen to their deliberations and learn what genetic engineering is achieving today and what is being planned in the areas of food production, pharmaceuticals, medicine, commerce, ecology, fuel efficiency, conservation, and so forth. I also heard about the government regulatory agencies and the very complex regulations with which they seek to oversee and control these developments.

Much of the scientific promise held out by this research had been summarized in an article by Fred Rosner, in which he points out that "medical science now has the capacity to rearrange the genetic heritage of thousands of years." He writes:

> Potential advantages of recombinant DNA research include: assembly of proteins valuable to man; insulin, antibiotics, antiviral agents and numerous other drugs, chemicals, and vaccines might be synthesized in large quantities by the technology of genetic engineering; patients with absent or defective genes suffering from such genetic disorders as Tay-Sachs disease, hemophilia, sickle cell anemia, and their like, might be given a replacement gene; nitrogen-producing bacteria for agriculture can be cloned; the supply of metals such as uranium and platinum might be increased by cloning bacteria that concentrate trace elements of such metals; pollution eating bacteria might be produced.[27]

---

27. Fred Rosner, "Genetic Engineering and Judaism," *Jewish Bioethics*, ed. Rosner and Bleich (Sanhedrin Press, 1979), pp. 409ff.

In fact, since Dr. Rosner's article was written, and while listening to the talks at the conference, I discovered that most of the above are already achieved, and much more besides.

For instance, the size of New York's refuse dump makes it visible to the naked eye from outer space. Genetically engineered bacteria can decompose and bio-degrade that dump and restore it to an environmentally friendly tract of land. Pollution from industry is being reduced, in one industry at the rate of ten percent per year, despite its ten percent annual growth, by genetic engineering.

Progress in medical research is proceeding as swiftly. HIV molecules, for instance, are too dangerous to handle, so in their effort to produce a vaccine, scientists are isolating various fractionate components of viruses that are immunogenic. Each isolated component is, by itself, safe. The component is made to reproduce and is expanded and purified, and vaccines are developed that are much safer than any which conventional bacteriology can produce. One of these experimental vaccines may yet be the answer to the threat of HIV, the AIDS virus.

Other developments involve traces of a certain protein that is produced deep in the human brain. This protein is needed for therapy of a fatal disease. Autopsy can produce a faint trace of this element, far too little to be of any use. Through genetic engineering it can be reproduced in sufficient quantity to render it useful in therapy. Then there is the leech, which does its business by sucking blood. It secretes a protein called hirudene that inhibits coagulation. By using a vector, transferring the genetic material by means of a virus, this protein can be injected into yeast, grown and expanded with the yeast, isolated, purified, and used in medicine as a very effective anti-coagulant. All this is only possible through genetic engineering techniques.

See also Goldstein, "Public Health Policy and Recombinant DNA," *New England Journal of Medicine* 296: (1977), pp. 1226–1228.

Unilever produces soap, biopharmaceuticals, diagnostics, and chemicals. In their measuring department, they have, through genetic engineering, developed processes that measure up to one unit of pollution—one molecule—in a liter of water, roughly equivalent to one gallon in Lake Michigan. In chemical production they have developed, through biotechnology, the ability to make many steps into one step, use low energy, low waste, benign instead of dangerous processes, new and renewable raw materials, and products so much cheaper that production costs of a certain precious and important chemical decreased from £864 a kilo to £24 a kilo.

But by far the most immediate effect for us is in the field of food production. In 1993 the Ministry of Agriculture, Food, and Fisheries asked specific questions and later requested a meeting with their Committee on Genetic Modification to discuss these issues. The Nuffield Foundation also asked similar questions. I shared my response with the members of the Chemical Industries Association.[28]

Finally, there remains the question of adequate control of these developments. There is no doubt that great harm can ensue from such genetic modification if not properly controlled.[29] An added element of danger is the fact that no country wants to require greater control than their competitors in trade, since that would place it at an economic disadvantage on the world market.

Cloning in man raises other moral and ethical issues. Vance Packard's *People Shapers* is no longer science fiction. Everywhere researchers are now considering the ethics and morals of this science. A National Bioethics Advisory Commission was appointed, studied the matter, and reported, and The Hastings

---

28. Supra, pp. xx, 14–20.
29. See Rosner, (supra, pp. 18f), who warns of enormous hazards of research going wrong and states that possibly worst of all is the fact that, once created, the new bugs cannot be destroyed.

Center has issued several articles in response.[30]

Lord Jakobovits' sentiments are expressed as follows:

> Without prior safeguards, there are no justifications for the experiments already undertaken in this sacred sphere, and a strict moratorium should be declared on further tests until the complex moral issues involved have been thoroughly examined, and some firm ethical guidelines are established to prevent abuses and excuses incompatible with the sanctity of life and its generation.
>
> It is indefensible to initiate controlled experiments with incalculable effects on the balance of nature and the preservation of man's incomparable spirituality without the most careful evaluation of the likely consequences beforehand.
>
> "Spare part" surgery and "genetic engineering" may open a wonderful chapter in the history of healing. But without prior agreement on restraints and the strictest limitations, such mechanization of human life may also herald irretrievable disaster resulting from man's encroachment upon nature's preserves, from assessing human beings by their potential value as tool-parts, sperm donors, or living incubators, and from replacing the matchless dignity of the human personality by test-tubes, syringes, and the soulless artificiality of computerized numbers.
>
> Man, as the delicately balanced fusion of body, mind, and soul, can never be the mere product of laboratory conditions and scientific ingenuity. To fulfill his destiny as a creative creature in the image of his Creator, he must be generated and reared out of the intimate love joining husband and wife together, out of identifiable parents who care for the development of their offspring, and out of a home which provides affectionate warmth and compassion.[31]

---

30. *The Hastings Center Report.* Volume 27, No. 5, September-October 1997.
31. Immanuel Jakobovits, *Eugenics in Jewish Medical Ethics*, Block Publishing Co., (New York, 1975), p. 261.

Rabbi Dr. Moshe D. Tendler cites similar objections and mentions the early experiments in human gene therapy, especially in the related field of in vitro fertilization.[32] Both Dr. Rosner and Rabbi Tendler conclude with Judaism's optimistic view of all such investigations, despite the hazards. The key issue is: is the intervention for therapy or for manipulation. Gene therapy can help cure dread diseases. Genetic manipulation "commodifies" man.[33]

---

32. Supra, pp. 21–25.
33. See also Azriel Rosenfeld, "Judaism and Gene Design," *Jewish Bioethics* pp. 401ff.

3

Sexuality and Reproduction

The questions dealt with almost every current issue concerning the beginning of life. They included queries about the Jewish attitude towards sexuality, homosexuality, birth control, conception, gender selection, procreation, abortion, embryo research, surrogacy, circumcision, infant's rights, and infant death. Following are selections of these questions and their answers.

Question: A woman has become a *Baalet Teshuva*, one who repents her past misdeeds. Previously, she had an ongoing relationship with a man who had two children by another woman. She often neglected contraception and yet did not become pregnant. There is nothing physiologically wrong with her, but she is now concerned lest she be infertile, and if so might find a *shiduch*, an appropriate marriage, problematical. Should she now have herself tested in order to ascertain the true state of affairs? It is well known that there are many causes of infertility that are temporary, and many more that are correctable. How far must she go in this matter?

Answer: I have checked with Rabbi Moshe Tendler on this matter. He had discussed such questions with his father-in-law, Rabbi Moshe Feinstein of blessed memory. Rabbi Feinstein's opinion is reflected in pertinent sections of the book *Practical Medical Halakhah.*[1]

She is definitely not required to investigate, and it would be unwise for her to do so. There could be many reasons why she did not conceive, not least of them the fact that she did not want to conceive and could have been avoiding her fertile period. In any case, while there is no outright prohibition against investigating her status of fertility, she is strongly advised not to do so. She should trust in God that in the merit of her return to observance a marriage into which she should enter would be blessed with children and with joy.[2]

---

1. Fred Rosner and Moshe D. Tendler, *Practical Medical Halakhah*, Third Edition (Ktav Publishing, 1990), p. 166. The discussion is about divulging an existent disability to a prospective spouse. It refers to a pre-existent condition, and the requirement is openness in the relationship between husband and wife. But the suspicion of a possible impediment or handicap when unfounded in fact and merely a conjecture, need not be divulged.
2. Rosner, in *Modern Medicine and Jewish Ethics*, has a chapter on screening for Tay-Sachs disease in which he stresses Rabbi Feinstein's concern for confidentiality. That requirement certainly applies in our case. See pp.161ff.

Sexuality

Question: What is the Jewish attitude towards pleasure in sex, and does it differ from the Christian attitude? Does Judaism consider partners equal during the act of sex and in the marriage bond? Does Judaism consider sex of value for its own sake, or only for the sake of procreation?

Answer: The primary purpose of the sex drive is, according to Judaism, to recreate the human race. Jewish law therefore severely limits contraception except for health considerations of the mother.[3] But it also accepts the pleasure of sex as God given, and one to be accepted with thanks to its Divine originator. It never considered sex to be evil or even merely an unfortunate necessity, as have some other faiths.[4]

---

3. Infra, p. 64f.
4. For a discussion of the approach of other faiths, see David M. Feldman, *Marital Relations, Birth Control and Abortion in Jewish Law*, (Shocken Books, New York 1975), pp. 21–27, 61–63, 83f. et passim.

It is good, as is every gift of God, but is to be regulated, as must be every gift of God. Sex is therefore forbidden outside of the marriage bond.

Judaism considers partners equal but different. Their differences must be taken into account, especially the different way they express their physical drives and needs. So the Jewish marriage contract requires that the husband satisfy the wife sexually, not the other way around. He must take her needs and desires into account, and may not, under any circumstances, force himself upon her. The sexual relationship is therefore in the woman's hands.

This is also expressed through the ritual of immersion in the ritual bath, or *mikvah*. Since the "biological clock" is built into the woman's physiology, it is she who, through this immersion, demonstrates her readiness for resuming the sexual relationship. Requiring this immersion as a religious obligation emphasizes the God-given quality of the gift of sex.

The prohibition of sexual relations from the onset of menstruation until seven days after its cessation is in keeping with the Divine origin of the gift of sex, for every physical appetite is limited in some way to demonstrate that we are not the masters, but the recipients of these gifts from the Master. Total liberty in any physical area indicates mastery. Limitation indicates that we are "borrowers" on this earth, and the Almighty is the true Master, the One who grants every gift we enjoy. By conforming to the ordained limits in the exercise of sex we acknowledge that the Almighty is the author of that gift.

Thus Rabbi Jacob Emden, a seventeenth-century sage, writes: "Sex in its proper circumstance—there is nothing better than that. In wrong circumstances, there is nothing worse."[5]

Nahmanides writes:

---

5. Rabbi Jacob Emden, Siddur Beit Ya'akov, Mittot Kesef 7, 33:17. (Lemberg ed.), p. 160.

The sexual act is holy and pure when carried on properly, in the proper time, and with the proper intentions. No one should claim that it is ugly or unseemly. God forbid! For intercourse is called "knowing" (Gen. 4:12) and not in vain is it called thus. . . . Understand that if marital intercourse did not partake of great holiness, it would not be called "knowing". . . . We do not believe that God created anything inherently ugly or unseemly. If we were to say that intercourse is repulsive then we blaspheme God who made the genitals . . . Hands can write a Sefer Torah and are then honorable and exalted. Hands too can perform evil deeds and then they are ugly. So [too] the genitals, . . . Whatever ugliness there is comes from how a person uses them. All organs of the body are neutral. The use made of them determines whether they are holy or unholy. . . .[6] Therefore, marital intercourse, under proper circumstances, is an exalted matter. . . . Now you can understand what our Rabbis meant when they declared, that when a husband unites with his wife in holiness, the Divine Presence is with them.[7]

There is a great deal of material available on this subject. I recommend *A Hedge of Roses* by Norman Lamm (Feldheim Publishers, New York, 1987); *Pardes Rimonim* by Moshe D. Tendler (Ktav Publishing, Hoboken, New Jersey, 1988), which deals mainly with Jewish "family purity laws"; *Jewish Medical Ethics* by Lord Immanuel Jakobovits (Bloch Publishing, New York); and *Jewish Bioethics* by Fred Rosner and J. David Bleich (Sanhedrin Press, New York, 1979), which has an entire section (pp. 59–197) on sexuality and procreation. Another excellent book is *Modern Medicine and Jewish Ethics* by Fred Rosner (Ktav Publishing, Hoboken, New Jersey, and

---

6. *Iggeret HaKodesh*, the "Epistle of Holiness," written to a friend on the subject of marriage. 176ff. Trans. by David Feldman loc. cit.
7. Talmud, *Sota* 17a.

Yeshiva University Press, New York, 1987) which has a section (pp. 75–173) on the beginning of life. In it you will find chapters on contraception, artificial insemination, in vitro fertilization, and much more. *Birth Control in Jewish Law* by David Feldman (New York University Press, New York, University of London Press, London, 1968) is a book devoted almost entirely to this subject.

Question: Does Judaism permit commitment of two partners outside of marriage, and what is the Jewish view about premarital sex? Is the Liberal Rabbi Brichto correct in his claim that Judaism does not condemn trial marriage, such as partners living together without marriage? Does not the Bible's advocacy of concubinage bear out his claim?

Answer: When Dr. Brichto's letter was printed in the London Times (June 39, 1991), I wrote the following letter in response, selections of which were published on July 6, 1991:

> Sir,
>
> Dr. Sidney Brichto speaks for himself but not for Judaism when he countenances premarital sexual relations and advocates for this purpose reinstating "betrothal," thus misunderstanding or misrepresenting that institution as Judaism practiced it.
>
> The "betrothal" to which Sidney Brichto alludes was a contractual engagement without sexual relations. It actually helped to keep the bride and groom inviolate before marriage, and to preserve their purity until the ceremony, as clearly indicated in such passages as Deuteronomy 22:23–28. That is why the Bible threatens the most severe penalty possible for sexual relations with a betrothed woman.
>
> Biblical as well as rabbinic sources require absolute abstinence from sex before marriage and total fidelity afterwards.

For example, Deuteronomy 23:18 forbidding prostitution and Leviticus 19:29 prohibiting immorality—warning that the land (society) would be corrupted otherwise—have always been taken in Jewish tradition to prohibit all manner of sexual relations outside of marriage. Such prohibitions are applied in rabbinic writings to both men and women.[8]

When Liberal Judaism, which Dr. Brichto represents, first appeared in Germany, its spokesmen claimed that they sought only to modify rituals and to eliminate observances which in their eyes seemed archaic. Thus they attacked synagogue forms, certain prayers, and the dietary laws. But they still insisted on holding sacred Judaism's moral code. Now Dr. Brichto attacks this same moral code, so basic to Jewish tradition, and seeks to do so in the name of Judaism.

The great majority of Jews in Britain belong to Orthodox synagogues and would feel deeply offended by Dr. Brichto's remarks. Judaism rejects tampering with religious precepts to suit immoral and dishonest times. It demands instead that we change the times we live in to conform to the standards taught by religion. The ideal of sexual abstinence till marriage and the purity and sacred nature of marriage itself is the bedrock upon which a sound and moral society is based. To undermine this ideal is to destroy the society we strive to preserve.

Question: What is the Jewish view concerning homosexuality? Does Judaism accept that some people may have an un-

---

8. Talmud, *Sanhedrin* 51, 82, *Berachot* 58. The prohibition of prostitution would in actual fact not strictly apply, since Judaism accepts marriage as possible by means of the sex act itself, though it is considered wrong and immoral to marry someone in this way. If, however, someone did marry by means of the sex act, then it is a full marriage and not a "trial marriage" at all, and Dr. Brichto's "betrothal" period certainly could not apply. See Maimonides *Mishneh Torah*, "Laws of Marriage" Chapter I, 1–4.

controllable drive towards homosexual practices and that there is likely to be a genetic basis for some of these propensities? Would Judaism consider someone to be sinful if he or she succumbed to homosexual propensities? Does it still hold him or her responsible even though this orientation might soon be proven to have a genetic base?

Answer: Lord Jakobovits was quoted by the newspapers (*London Jewish Chronicle*, and *London Times* of July 17, 1993) as saying that if it can be shown that there is a genetic propensity to homosexuality, then this orientation can be considered an illness and not a natural condition. Treatment for such a condition, if available, would not be a violation of Jewish tradition.

There was a strong negative reaction to this from the homosexual lobby. Lord Jakobovits was accused of proposing a Nazi-like "solution" and it was claimed that we were embarking on a program resembling Hitler's policy of forced sterilization. Newspapers began to call the Chief Rabbi's office. Lord Jakobovits suggested I write to clarify his misquoted views. I did so. The newspapers, after printing the letter, called me and misquoted me as well. Finally, I prepared a letter to answer the accusations and to clarify Judaism's view. It was, however, felt that the furor was dying down, and that the second letter should be withheld for the moment. Following is the first letter I wrote to explain the stand Judaism takes as enunciated by Lord Jakobovits in the London *Times*. It was printed on July 27, 1993:

Sir,

The recently publicized views (report July 16) that proneness to homosexuality may be genetically transmitted has given rise to a stormy response. Judaism has a definite view, clearly and succinctly expressed by Lord Jakobovits in his letter to your newspaper (July 17). I am saddened by the intolerance of his detractors, prepared to stoop to obscene comparison with Nazi extermination (letters July 20).

To Judaism, abhorrence of homosexual conduct is altogether compatible with sympathy for homosexuals, especially since they may expose themselves and others to a hideous contagion.

Judaism believes that we must be masters of human nature, not enslaved by it. For some, it may be more difficult to control their nature and resist its drives than for others. God's law remains in force, whether harder or easier to follow.

Cain was not merely informed that sin crouches at the door. He was also told that it would draw him on with a magnetic power of attraction. He was commanded to resist that power and to master his inclination.

The Bible considers homosexuality to be an abomination, one of the most severe transgressions of God's Law. Society, by condoning it, has made it all the harder to resist. But resist we must, however we are inclined, whether the inclination is genetic, social, psychological, or simply the result of "the pleasure of being contrary."

It is particularly painful that some dissident Jewish spokesmen, having abandoned many Jewish religious observances long ago, should now publicly denounce basic Jewish moral teachings enshrined in Biblical law.[9]

---

9. The expected polemic ensued in letters to me and to the *Times*. Following are samples of the comments, pro and con: "How glad I was to read Rabbi Shulman's letter today. It is not often that true morality is allowed voice—and Biblical authority to support it. He put it so well and clearly that it reminded me that the contribution of the Jewish people to the world is primarily a *moral force*," and on the other hand: "I am Jewish, homosexual, and happy. Is it any wonder that you and Lord Jakobovits have the dubious privilege of presiding over an era in which Jews are abandoning their religion in droves, when faced with this kind of teaching? Kindly remember that in some cultures it is an abhorrence to be Jewish." The polemic became so heated that newspapers pursued me to New Zealand, where I was enjoying a quiet holiday with my wife.

Following is part of the text of the subsequent letter that I proposed but that was never sent, since the tumult had subsided:

> While genetic engineering to correct "gene grouping defects" is at present still in the realm of science fiction, the Bible classification of homosexuality as one of the most severe transgressions is clear. Every means must be pursued to overcome tendencies and inclinations towards this transgression. Judaism strongly believes that man must master his nature, not be enslaved by it. Psychological, social or even genetic propensities notwithstanding, homosexual conduct is forbidden. If "gene grouping defects" are ever in the future correctable, and if a person approaches a religious Jewish doctor seeking such correction, the doctor would be perfectly within the mandate of Judaism to help such a patient medically.

Finally, I received a letter from David Shapiro, Executive Secretary of the Nuffield Council of Bioethics, in which he stated: "I should really have guessed that the newspapers had managed to quote you out of context in the great fuss about the so-called 'homosexuality gene.' We must give thanks that that particular fuss has died away for the moment. No doubt it will recur. Next time let us hope that the journalists can be got to read the original article and focus their questions more sensibly."

Question: I am writing a book on views toward sex as reflected by various religious groups. I have come across a polemic between Rabbi Meiselman, who declares that morality and fidelity are basic ingredients of Jewish marriage and that the partners are each given full consideration, and Rachel Biale, who points to Biblical polygamy and Jewish permissiveness towards concubinage to indicate that Judaism's view of marriage is sorely out of date. Indeed, the Biblical narratives seem to bear out Rachel Biale's point of view, indicating that adultery was a one-way street, and that only a woman would be branded as an adulteress, but not a man who had relations with another woman, provided she be unmarried. I am further confused by Dr. Brichto's advocacy of trial marriage, which would indicate that sexual morality is not high on the scale in Jewish marriage values and in Jewish attitudes. Yet I read your statement in the *Times* that indicates you are in agreement with Rabbi Meiselman. Can you respond, please.

Answer: I wish you great success in your forthcoming book. Perhaps the following comments might help. But first, allow me to correct an error in your question. In Judaism's view an unmarried woman is *not* an adulteress.

Rabbi Moshe Meiselman writes with a clear perception of what Jewish law requires. Traditional Judaism is based on the Bible and the oral tradition that has been transmitted through the centuries by the Jewish people through their study and especially by the unbroken tradition of rabbinic teaching. It is not possible to understand what Judaism requires without linking the written and the oral tradition together. For that reason Rachel Biale does not capture the spirit of Judaism, while Rabbi Meiselman does.

If you read some of the Bible verses without a notion of how Judaism understands and interprets them, you might well come to the view that Rachel Biale has. A more detailed study of the verses concerned, however, will point to the likelihood that the rabbinic interpretation is really the simple intent of the passages.

I shall offer below a few verses of the Torah with the explanatory rabbinic teaching. But before I do so, a word must be said about polygamy.

We cannot judge yesterday by today. Nowadays monogamy is the rule. Once upon a time the rule was polygamy. Even so, the Bible obviously discouraged polygamy. Abraham and Isaac were monogamous. Jacob would have also been monogamous, were he not tricked into a marriage with Rachel's older sister and later required by his two wives to marry their handmaids in order to help them in their childbearing rivalry. All of this took place before the Mount Sinai experience when our people received the Torah. Once the Torah was given, the rules became more rigid, and sisters were not permitted to marry the same man. Polygamy continued. It was the rabbis, and particularly Rabbenu Gershom of the tenth-century Franco–German Empire, who outlawed polygamy because we were living among people who were monogamous. In those areas of the world where polygamy continued, Jews have not been required to live monogamously even until this very day. Even so, the spirit of the patriarchs infused our people to the extent that you do not find any of the rabbis of the Mishnah and Talmud who had more than one wife. Apparently, monogamy was in practice with few exceptions even during a period of time when polygamy was theoretically permitted.

In a polygamous society, if a husband has relations with an unmarried woman, it can obviously be construed that she is, or becomes, a second wife, while if a married woman has relations with another man she is committing a forbidden act. Insofar as this is the case, Miss Biale is correct. Adultery therefore becomes defined as a wife having sex with another man outside of her marriage, or a man having sex with a married woman.

As for concubines, the only difference in Jewish law between a concubine and a wife is the requirement that in case of divorce or widowhood, the husband must provide a stated amount of support called *ketuvah* to a wife, while most authorities do not require this for concubines. Some rabbinic authorities do require it for concubines as well.[10]

---

10. *Pilegesh*, commonly translated "concubine," is actually better translated as "common-law wife." Jewish law uses the term for a relationship where a woman is dedicated to a man without the benefit of the marriage ceremony. Maimonides, on the

There is an interesting principle of Jewish law that is based on the moral conduct of the Jewish community, namely that "a man does not have intercourse for reasons of sexual promiscuity, but has in mind marriage, unless otherwise indicated." To put it more simply: Judaism recognises two partners who have sex as being married in common law. Thus, if a man has sex with an unmarried woman, it is assumed to be for the sake of marriage. She is then considered his wife. The rabbis thought this was a nasty way to get married and discouraged it, but acknowledged the validity of such a common law marriage. On the other hand, if it is clear that the partners simply meant to have a casual relationship, then this is construed by many to be the *zenut*, "prostitution," of which the Torah speaks when it condemns male and female prostitution.

I would suggest that it must be either/or. Either a man is absolutely forbidden to have casual sex by Torah decree, or casual sex does not exist because it creates a marriage arrangement. You cannot have it both ways.

I shall now cite a few verses of the Torah with rabbinic comments, referring especially to Maimonides' Code upon which subsequent codes of Jewish law are based. I do so in order to help you sense the meaning of Bible verses as our rabbis understood them, and to make you aware of why they perceived in these verses a clear demand for total abstinence outside of marriage.

"There shall not be a male or female prostitute..." (Deuteronomy 23:18). Do not think this refers only to a professional prostitute. The rabbis define *kedesha* as someone with whom a person has casual sex—cohabiting without a

---

basis of the Talmud (*Sanhedrin* 21a), rules that a *pilegesh* lacks the formal bonds of marriage and the ceremony and the security of the *ketuvah*. Rashi rules that she does have formal bonds of marriage even without the ceremony and lacks only the *ketuvah*. Rashi's view is borne out by a passage in the Jerusalem Talmud (Ketuvot I:2).

ketuvah and without a marriage ceremony. Rabbi Joseph Babad, in his code of Torah commandments, *Minchat Hinuch*, summarizes the general rabbinic view as follows: "We are prohibited to cohabit with a woman without a marriage contract and a proper ceremony of marriage, and that is the meaning of 'There shall not be a male or female prostitute...' (Deuteronomy 23:18)"[11] And Maimonides explains: "The Torah emphasizes this commandment by repeating 'Thou shalt not defile your daughter to allow her to prostitute herself'" *Sifre* (an early halakhic exegetical commentary on the Bible) notes: "'Thou shalt not defile your daughter' refers to a person who gives his daughter [to a man] for sex without marriage, and so too if she gives herself to a man for this purpose."[12]

Maimonides, in his listing and explanation of Torah commandments, adds that we are forbidden to cohabit "except through marriage, by means of a contract of marriage, or a transaction creating the marriage bond, or through a sexual act which creates the marriage bond, and this is the essence of the commandment of *kiddushin*. Therefore the Torah [Deut. 24:1] declared, 'When a man takes a wife and cohabits with her...' "[13]

Maimonides infers from these and other such verses that "[i]f someone cohabits with a woman, casually ['in the spirit of harlotry'], he is permitted by Torah law to marry any of her relatives, but the Rabbis prohibited this [to the seven degrees of consanguinity] as long as the harlot [the woman with whom he had casual sex] is alive, since she visits her relatives and the proximity and familiarity may cause him to sin again."[14]

---

11. Rabbi Joseph Babad, *Sefer HaHinuch*, Commandment 357.
12. Maimonides, *Book of Commandments*, "Prohibitions," no. 355.
13. Maimonides, *Book of Commandments*, "Positive Commandments," no. 213.
14. Maimonides, *Mishneh Torah*, Laws of Forbidden Sex, Ch. II, no. 11.

I also refer you to the Talmud *Sanhedrin* 105–106, which describes the evil council Balaam gave to Balak that caused Balak to try to entice the Jews away from God by letting loose a band of beautiful prostitutes: "Their God hates immorality, so. . . ." In the ensuing episode in the Bible Pinchas slays the sinning prince of Israel together with the prostitute (Numbers 25:7–9). She was actually, according to the Bible testimony (Numbers 25:15), a Midianite princess.

Apparently the Bible sometimes calls anyone engaging in immoral practice a "prostitute." This is borne out by Maimonides' statement interpreting the word with a much larger scope than we usually attribute to it, indicating that it includes, according to the oral tradition, such women as we are forbidden to marry by Torah law, such as a married woman, one forbidden by consanguinity, or a non-Jewess, and so forth. He then indicates that, while engaging in casual sex with a woman we are actually permitted to marry does not precisely render her a prostitute, nevertheless it merits the penalty of lashes.[15] He also states that "One is permitted to look at a woman's face to determine if she is good-looking in order to decide whether to ask her to marry him, but he may not look at her with a lascivious eye."[16]

These are but a few of the countless sources that all point in the same direction. It is inconceivable that Dr. Brichto did not know at least some of them. His error is in discarding the oral tradition, reading the written tradition very literally and fundamentally, and, finally, imposing the standards of morality we find today on the previous generations.

The effect of the Biblical laws as interpreted by the rabbis was such that for most of Jewish history a very moral society was created. I would like to refer you to three books that deal with morality in the Jewish community in the Middle Ages and thereafter. They do not glorify the moral standards of the

15. Ibid., Ch. XVIII, Nos. 1, 2.
16. Maimonides, Ibid, Ch. XXI, No. 3.

Jewish community but indicate the exceptions as well as the rule. They are Dr. Irving Agus, *The Heroic Age of Franco-German Jewry*, (Yeshiva University Press, New York, 1969); *Urban Civilization in Pre-Crusade Europe* (2 volumes) by the same author, Dr. Irving Agus, (Yeshiva University Press, New York, 1965); and part of a chapter in my own book, *Authority and Community 16th Century Polish Jewry* (Yeshiva University Press and Ktav, Hoboken, N.J., 1986). Indexes and tables of contents in each case will indicate where you should look. The second and third books deal specifically with questions of morality. The third also deals with polygamy.

Birth Control

Question: How does Judaism view contraceptives, coitus interruptus, and other forms of birth control? An article in the medical journal *The General Practitioner* by Deborah Wilcox[17] seems to indicate Judaism has permissive views about such matters. Is this true? Is her claim that Jewish husbands must cohabit with their wives on Friday night true?

Answer: Deborah Wilcox's article is inaccurate and misleading. Her statement about Friday night is false. Lionel Kopelowitz, M.D., former President of the Board of Deputies of British Jews, joined me in framing an answer to that article.[18] Our joint statement is as follows:

Sir,

We have read the article "Religion Affects Birth Control" by Deborah Wilcox. Her references to Judaism are totally inac-

---

17. November 26, 1993, pp. 56ff.
18. *The General Practitioner* did not publish our statement.

63

curate and grossly misleading.

Judaism lists the duty of procreation ("Be fruitful and multiply," *Gen.* 1:28; 9:1) as the first commandment of the Torah. Conversely, it deems the pointless destruction of the human seed to be a grave violation of this obligation.[19]

Contraception is therefore prohibited, except when overridden by considerations of the mother's health.[20] The *Compendium of Jewish Medical Ethics*, published by the Jewish Medical Ethics, of New York, summarizes the Jewish view as follows:

> Contraceptive devices may not be used except [when demanded by health considerations]. Contraception . . . is incompatible with the Jewish emphasis on procreation. When medical indications . . . necessitate the practice of birth control, Jewish law grades the contraceptive techniques from least to most objectionable in the following order: oral contraceptives, chemical spermicides, diaphragms and cervical caps to be used by the wife, and condoms. The least objectionable should be used when contraception is medically required.[21]

Ms. Wilcox's statement that a husband must cohabit on Friday night is nonsense. Judaism includes in the marriage con-

---

19. Rabbi Joseph Babad, *Sefer HaHinukh*, a fourteenth-century listing and explanation of commandments, lists this commandment as first in the order of importance: "The purpose of this commandment is that the world be populated. It is a great *mitzvah*, for, through it, all other commandments . . . may be fulfilled" (*Mitzvah* No. 1). Destruction of seed (semen) for no cause was a great sin, and was understood to be the reason Onan was killed by the Almighty (Gen. 38:7–10). Maimonides states: "It is forbidden to expend semen to no purpose" (*Mishneh Torah*, "Laws of Prohibited Sexual Relations," 21:18).
20. *Talmud Yevamot*, 12b. Maimonides, *Mishneh Torah*, Hilchot Issurei Bi'a 12:12. *Code of Jewish Law*, Even Ha'ezer 5:12.
21. *Compendium on Medical Ethics* (New York 1984), p. 45f.

tract the requirement that the husband must satisfy his wife sexually, not the other way around. Some sages indicated that sexual pleasure on Friday night can enhance the joy of the Sabbath, but they in no way required it.[22]

Coitus interruptus is banned in Judaism. The Compendium discusses the medical investigation of a sterility problem when it is necessary to test the semen for quantity and quality of sperm. Though the condom or interrupted coitus are not ordinarily permitted by Jewish law, yet when the intent of the act is to fulfil the obligation to have children and to satisfy the couple's otherwise unattainable desire to do so, the use of these methods may be considered for collecting and testing sperm. This should be done in consultation with Rabbinic authority. Under those circumstances, and by medical indication only, Rabbinic opinion may permit even more lenient methods of semen collection.

Question: What does Judaism say about the dangers of world overpopulation? Considering how population grows far faster than food supply, is it not compassionate to advocate birth control? Is not the Chinese formula for limitation of birth worth adopting by the Western world?

Answer: I read your words with interest and suggest that, in considering this question, you have overlooked the most important element of all, the element of freedom. China denies human rights in its birth control program. Any program

22. Rabbi Isaac Aboab, *Menorat HaMaor*, Ner III, Klal VI, part V, Ch. 3 (Mosad Harav Kook), p. 390: "One should not intend his own pleasure alone—but his wife's as well," and the *Book of the Pious* of the thirteenth century in the same vein at greater length. A number of such sources are collected by D. Feldman op. cit., Ch. 9–13.

the world might mount must be optional for the participants, for otherwise such a program would be tantamount to enslavement, forbidden by Jewish as well as humanitarian law.

Food production does keep up with the population, the Malthusian theory notwithstanding. Future generations will have to find still more imaginative ways to feed the world's population, and they can.

Most people do not consider that the commandment "Be fruitful and multiply" applies nowadays as it always has. We consider this a required command, at least for Jews. Is it required for others? That is a matter discussed by the rabbis and in which there is divergent opinion. (As you may know, the requirement to be fruitful is satisfied, according to most authorities, when a boy and girl are born, symbolic of the continuation of the race.)

What are the facts? Jews are, unfortunately, doing far more than their share to limit the growth of population. We have the lowest birthrate of any group in the Western world. We compound this low rate—not enough to maintain anywhere near our present numbers—with a very high rate of assimilation, well over fifty percent in America, close to forty percent in Britain, and further compound it with an astonishingly high abortion rate in Israel as well as elsewhere in Jewish communities worldwide. I consider this to be a form of racial suicide and feel no obligation to the rest of the planet, especially since we are underpopulating while they are overpopulating, and more especially after Hitler's program of genocide destroyed one-third of the Jewish people.

In Vitro Fertilization, Conception, Procreation, and Gender Selection

Question: What is the Jewish position regarding in vitro fertilization for infertile couples? I have spoken to representatives of some of the pro-life organizations as well as of the Roman Catholic Church, the Church of England, and the Methodist Church.

Answer: Judaism does not consider infertility to be a condition that one must accept without making efforts to reverse or change it. Judaism requires medical intervention to cure illness, for there is a divine mandate to heal the sick. In the same way Judaism encourages medical intervention in the effort to cure infertility, for Judaism places infertility in the category of illness. As with all illness, some risk may be undertaken during treatment to secure the large gain of health, in this case renewed fertility.

Following is an excerpt, with minor revisions, from an article I wrote on this subject which will further clarify this matter:

The Beginning of Life: The Jewish Point of View

Science has broken through many barriers in its attempt to combat infertility and help conception. Not everyone agrees that this is a good thing. Some faith communities have made a virtue of the natural, the unnatural being unclean or unholy. But Judaism maintains that the human being is given a task on earth to use nature for his benefit, and a responsibility to nurture and protect it, for he is a steward of the Almighty. For the world was purposely created with imperfections so that man can join with Almighty God in perfecting this world. In so doing, he becomes a partner with God in creation. Among his most important mandates is to heal the sick.

It would seem that helping fertilization is totally in keeping with this point of view. But this is not so simple. For birth techniques pose some risks. The procurement of the egg by means of laparoscopy involves a small risk of medical and surgical complications. Jewish law forbids a person to incur injury except in pursuit of therapeutic benefit. It must therefore first be determined whether in vitro fertilization is in the category of therapy. If it is, then risks and benefits can be weighed to determine whether the procedure may be used.

Judaism points to the pain of the Patriarchs who were barren—especially Rachel, who cried out in anguish, "Give me children, else I die" (Gen. 30:1), to demonstrate that sterility, although not life threatening, may cause psychic trauma to a childless couple who desperately desire a child, be it for personal fulfilment or for social or religious obligations. This places sterility in the category of illness. So Judaism considers intervention in birth techniques a legitimate way to treat a condition of barrenness. The many rules and guidelines that govern what may and may not be done to cure illness apply to this area as well.[23]

---

23. Shulman, *Australia and New Zealand Jewish Year Book, Bicentennial Edition*, ed. Jacqueline Langley (York Press, Abbotsford, Victoria, 1988), pp. 85ff.

Fertility Medicine

Questions: I am a student at Queensferry High School doing an investigation in Religious Studies about "manipulating nature." I am particularly interested in receiving information with regard to test tube babies, surrogacy, sex selection, and abortion. . . .

As a third-year law student at the University of Westminster, I am embarking on a Philosophy of Law dissertation on "Fertility, Medicine, and the Law." I would like to include the view Judaism takes concerning these matters. . . .

I am currently writing a book on culture, religion, and childbearing. I would like the Jewish perspective on contraception, infertility, miscarriage, screening for fetal abnormality, termination of pregnancy, prematurity, and stillbirth.

Answer: Following is a slightly revised version of an article I wrote on the subject, which was published in Australia:[24]

The Beginning of Life: The Jewish Point of View

The Vatican position on the beginning of life, which appeared more than ten years ago under the title "Instruction on Respect for Human Life in its Origin and on the Dignity of Procreation," gave the Catholic view of issues that are at the base of our understanding of life, the embryo, the purpose and the act of conjugal sex, the family, the relationship of man to nature, and in fact the future of society itself. The Protestant community has its own point of view, not at all uniform.[25] Parliament has also debated this issue.

---

24. Ibid., pp. 82–88.
25. The most important non-sectarian group involved in ethical analysis of such questions is probably The Hastings Institute in Hastings-on-Hudson, New York, a nonprofit, nonpartisan organization that carries out educational and research programs on

The Jewish point of view in this debate is immensely important, because Judaism has dealt with these questions from the time of their first appearance on the scene; because there are groups within Judaism that have made it their exclusive business to study these and other questions of medical ethics from the Jewish point of view; and because the Jewish point of view is based on Judaism's worldview which is very old, and which addresses many of these questions from a very different perspective than does the Catholic and the Protestant Church. Jewish thought and law have a very large contribution to make towards resolving these important and difficult issues. The main principles upon which Judaism bases many of its decisions concerning the beginning of life, include the following:

Human life is infinitely important. The Bible is at pains to describe all people of the world as descended from one human, to emphasize that each person can populate an entire world. Every human being, whole or impaired, perfect or deformed, has a full right and a full claim on life and all that society can do to preserve that life. One cannot consider a defect in the quality or quantity of life as a valid reason for diminishing the claim of that individual on society's protection of his life. Since human life is of infinite importance, no one can say, "My life is more important than yours." Each person can reply to his neighbor, "Are we not all equal? After all, we are equally descended from the same person."[26] Nevertheless, if one person is a pursuer of another with intent to kill, the intended victim is given precedence, so the person who seeks to end another's life forfeits his own, if that is the only way to save the victim from his attacker.

The family is the most important and sacred unit of society. Judaism creates certain restrictions to safeguard the sanc-

---

ethical issues in medicine, the life sciences, and the professions. They publish a periodical called *The Hastings Report.*
26. Talmud, *Sanhedrin* 37a.

tity of the family, while demanding of man that he create a family, procreate, and provide for future generations.

Man is given a task on earth to use nature for his benefit, and a responsibility to nurture and protect it as a steward of the Almighty. The world was purposely created with imperfections so that man can join with Almighty God in perfecting this world, and in so doing, he becomes a partner with God in creation. Thus man must advance with the advance of science. He builds bridges, conquers floods, develops new methods of irrigation, manufacture, and creative art. He crosses oceans and creates machines that conquer the air and ultimately the far reaches of space. In all this he conquers, uses, and even changes the natural world. And among his most important mandates is to heal the sick. For Judaism does not believe that naturalness is necessarily a virtue:

> Although we are required to respect and care for God's creation, we are also required to build upon what we are given and improve upon creation. For the world was created purposely imperfect so that man may join with God in perfecting it. Rabbi Akiva taught this lesson to the Roman tyrant Tinneius Rufus who's philosophy was to maintain the status quo (*supra*, p. 29). Only if we consider man's greatest *mitzvah* to join with God in the sacred act of creation, can we regard the artificial heart, artificial kidney and artificial insemination as a great good deed of a physician.[27]

Additional principles that are relevant include the following:

Judaism lists the duty of procreation ("Be fruitful and multiply," Gen. 1:28; 9:1) as the first of its 613 Commandments.[28] Conversely, it deems the pointless destruction of the human seed as a grave violation of this law.[29]

---

27. Moshe D. Tendler, "Rabbinic Comment: Transplantation Surgery," *The Mount Sinai Journal of Medicine*, Vol. 51, No. 1 (New York, January-February 1984), p. 54; see supra, p. 11.
28. *Shulhan Aruch* (Code of Jewish Law), *Even Haezer*, I:1.
29. Ibid., XXIII.

Judaism's strict code of sexual morality, especially the laws on incest (Leviticus 18:1–30; 20:8–27), presupposes that the (biological) father and mother of a child are known and can be identified with absolute certainty. No legal contract or artificial act can suspend, override, or replace natural relationships based on consanguinity.[30]

The duty to preserve human life and health is a religious precept[31] that includes the divine sanction of intervention in the course of nature or providence by the practice of medicine.[32] But this sanction conferred on doctors is limited to acts of healing or procedures intended to serve therapeutic ends.

Man, created to "hold dominion over the fish of the sea and the birds of the air and every living thing crawling on the earth," [33] is entitled to exploit animals in his service and for his health, provided they are protected from all avoidable suffering. He is, however, forbidden deliberately to mix diverse living species[34]

Abortion

The Catholic view is that abortion is worse than murder, because murder kills only the body, while abortion condemns the eternal soul, for the fetus is not yet baptized.[35] It is therefore never permitted, even if the mother's life is at risk. St.

30. See Rabbis Abraham Akiva Rodner, Moshe Findelberg and B. M. Mizrachi for a discussion of the legal quality of adoption according to Jewish law and for a discussion of the ruling that biological legal fictions cannot be set up. *Noam*, Vol. IV, (Jerusalem 1960), pp. 61–145.
31. *Deuteronomy*, 4:9, 15.
32. *Exodus*, 21:19.
33. *Genesis*, 1:28.
34. *Leviticus*, 19:19, Genesis, 1:11, 12, 21, 25. See Jakobovits, loc. cit.
35. E. F. Healy, *Medical Ethics* (Chicago: Loyola University Press, 1956), pp. 357f.; J. Marshall, *The Ethics of Medical Practice* (London: Darton Longman and Todd, 1960), pp. 152f.

Augustine and other early Christian authorities maintained that the unborn child was included among those condemned to eternal perdition if it died unbaptized.[36] On 29 October 1951, Pope Pius XII delivered an address on morality in marriage in which he stated:

> Every human being, even the infant in its mother's womb, has the right to life immediately from God. . . . Therefore, there is no man, no human authority, no science, no medical, eugenic, social, economic, or moral indication, that can show or give valid juridicial title for direct deliberate disposition concerning an innocent life. . . . Thus, for example, to save the life of the mother is a most noble end, but the direct killing of the child as a means to this end is not licit.[37]

This position is maintained till this present day. It has been strongly restated in the Vatican document on procreation.[38]

What is the Jewish view? In the Jewish view abortion is not permitted because it is the killing of potential life and can therefore be sanctioned only for a correspondingly grave hazard to the life or health of the mother. The hazards are ordinarily physical, but can include psychiatric disturbances caused or aggravated by the continued pregnancy, or anguish expressed as suicidal tendencies. Under such conditions an abortion is mandated, since the life and well-being of the mother take priority over that of her unborn child.[39] We do not believe in original sin, or that man is born tainted. The newborn is pure, and we do not worry about its entering heaven.

---

36. Ploss and Bartels, *Woman* (1925) p. 483; *Catholic Encyclopedia*, (1907), pp. 266f., 923ff., Catholic Hospital Association of the United States and Canada, *Ethical and Religious Directives for Catholic Hospitals*, (1949), p. 4.
37. C. Y. McFadden, *Medical Ethics*, 5th edition, (Philadelphia: F. A. Davis Co., 1961) pp. 140f.
38. Ibid.
39. *Compendium*, p. 49.

Fetal indications, such as fear of deformity because of the mother's exposure to rubella or other viral diseases, or because drugs may have affected fetal development, do not in themselves justify recourse to abortion. Generally, indications must be maternal rather than fetal. As Rabbi Jakobovits states:

> All the authorities of Jewish law are agreed that physical or mental abnormalities do not in themselves compromise the title to life, whether before or after birth. Cripples and idiots, however incapacitated, enjoy the same human rights (though not necessarily legal competence) as normal persons.[40] An idiot can even sue for personal injuries inflicted on him.[41] The killing of even a dying person is culpable as murder.[42] Since human life is of infinite value, its sanctity is bound to be entirely unaffected by the absence of any or all mental faculties or by any bodily defects: any fraction of infinity still remains infinite.[43]

Some authorities, among them the Israeli sages Rabbi Eliezer Waldenberg and the late Rabbi Shaul Yisraeli, are quite lenient in considering maternal psychological harm as cause for abortion, especially when considered during the first ninety days of pregnancy. They even permit termination in some cases where the pregnancy is detrimental to the mother's health, even though not actually life-threatening, provided that no fetal movement has as yet been felt.[44] These opinions were

---

40. "Biur Halakhah" on *Mishnah Berurah Shulchan Aruch, Orah Hayyim* 329:4.
41. Talmud, Baba Kamma 8:4.
42. Maimonides, *Mishneh Torah*, "*Hilkhot Roze'ah*" 2:7.
43. Immanuel Jakobovits, "Jewish Views on Abortion" *Jewish Bioethics*, ed. Rosner and Bleich, (Sanhedrin Press, New York, 1979), p. 123.
44. Shaul Yisraeli, *Amud HaYemini*, No. 32; Eliezer Waldenberg, *Tzitz Eliezer* Vol. III (Jerusalem, 5723), No. 48, p. 190; Vol. VIII (Jerusalem, 5725), No. 36, pp. 218f., and Vol. IX (Jerusalem, 5727), No. 51, pp. 233–240; J. David Bleich, *Contempo-*

rejected by Rabbi Moshe Feinstein who considers them not to be in consonance with Jewish law. He would prohibit abortion unless the mother is suicidal, or otherwise severely disturbed.[45]

There is halakhic basis for a difference in approach to abortion between the first forty days of pregnancy and afterwards, since abortion during this first forty-day period is performed on a relatively unformed embryo. After forty days, abortion is considered killing, although it is not punishable by death in Jewish law.[46] Authorities agree that it is to be considered at least the taking of "potential life."[47] In all cases where an abortion is being considered, rabbinic authority must be consulted.

The Family and Procreation

Judaism requires man to do all in his power to enable children to be born to couples who would otherwise be childless, consistent with morality and *halakhah*. Various methods of coping with infertility must therefore be considered.

Artificial Insemination

a. Donor Sperm. Jewish religious law usually forbids this type of insemination, since it presents a practical question about

rary Halakhic Problems, (New York, 1977), pp. 112–115, and Samuel Hayyim Katz, *HaPardes*, Tamuz 5735. See also Rosner and Bleich Jewish Bioethics, pp. 138, 146, and nn. 10 and 46.

45. Moshe Feinstein, *Iggros Moshe*, "Hoshen Mishpat Part II", No. 69. That responsum speaks only of the possibility of self-harm. Orally, in a conversation reported to me by Dr. Melvin Zelefsky who had been his student, the danger of potential bodily mortal harm to the newborn child was mentioned.

46. J. David Bleich, "Abortion in Halakhic Literature," *Jewish Bioethics*, pp. 142–146.

47. Moshe D. Tendler, "Population Control, the Jewish Point of View," Jewish Bioethics, p. 101. Immanuel Jakobovits, *"Jewish Views on Abortion,"* op. cit., p. 120.

the actual paternity of such a child and creates the possibility of subsequent incestuous unions among children fathered by the same donor. Nevertheless, there is no stigma of illegitimacy attached to any child born in such a way.[48]

b. Husband's Sperm: This is to be considered part of the total management of an infertile couple and is permitted.[49]

c. Sperm Banks: The eugenic considerations proposed for sperm banks, in which genetically "superior" sperm is stored, run contrary to the philosophy and spirit of Judaism. Sperm bank projects for this purpose are to be discouraged with vigor, since they unnecessarily compromise the human dimension of life and family.[50]

An excellent summary of Jewish views on this subject is given by Dr. Fred Rosner:

> Artificial insemination using the semen of a donor other than the husband is considered by most rabbinic opinion to be an abomination and strictly prohibited for a variety of reasons, including the possibility of incest, lack of genealogy, and the problems of inheritance. Some authorities regard A.I.D. (Artificial Insemination, Donor) as adultery, requiring the husband to divorce his wife and her forfeiture of the *ketubah*, and even the physician and the donor are guilty when involved in this act akin to adultery. Most rabbinic opinion, however, holds that unless a sexual act is involved, the woman is not guilty of adultery and is not prohibited subsequently to cohabit with her husband. Nor is there any stigma of bastardy to the offspring.

---

48. For a short discussion of both sides of this issue, see J. David Bleich, "Survey of Recent Halakhic Periodic Literature," *Tradition*, Vol. 32 No. 2, Winter 1998 (Rabbinical Council of America, New York), ed. Emanuel Feldman, pp. 152f. The prevailing view that the child bears no stigma of bastardy is discussed by Rabbi Moshe Feinstein, *Iggros Moshe Even Haezer* (New York 1951–1961), I:10, 71, III:14.
49. See Rabbi Feinstein, Ibid.
50. See Rabbi Jakobovits, *loc. cit.*, and *Compendium* p. 49.

Regarding the status of the child, rabbinic opinion is divided. Most consider the offspring to be legitimate.... Considerable rabbinic opinion regards the child to be the son of the donor in all respects (*i.e.*, inheritance, support, custody, incest... and the like).

There is near unanimity of opinion that the use of semen from the husband is permissible if no other method is possible for the wife to become pregnant. However, certain qualifications exist. Most authorities require a reasonable period of waiting since marriage (... or until medical proof of the absolute necessity for A.I.H.), and, according to many authorities, the insemination may not be performed during the wife's period of ritual impurity. It is permitted by most rabbis to obtain sperm from the husband both for analysis and for insemination, but difference of opinion exists as to the method to be used in the procurement of it. Masturbation should be avoided if possible, and coitus interruptus, retrieval of sperm from the vagina, or the use of a condom seem to be the preferred methods.[51]

In Vitro Fertilization

a. Maternal risk factors. The procurement of the egg by means of laparoscopy involves a small risk of medical and surgical complications. Jewish law forbids persons to injure themselves except in pursuit of therapeutic benefit. It must therefore first be determined that IVF is in the category of therapy. If so, then risks and benefits must be weighed to determine whether the procedure may be used. If there were no risks at all to the patient, then there would be no question that such procedures would be permissible. If risks exist with little or no benefit, then the prohibition against self-mutilation and self-harm would prohibit such procedures.

---

51. F. Rosner, "Artificial Insemination in Jewish Law," *Jewish Bioethics*, pp. 115f.

Sterility (barrenness), although not life threatening, may cause psychic trauma to a childless couple who desperately desire a child, be it for personal fulfilment or for social or religious obligations. This fact places sterility in the category of illness and justifies assuming the risk of laparoscopy and/ or hormonal treatment.[52] A married couple who wish to become parents would have justifiable reasons to undertake the minimum risk involved. The patient's decision making is dominant in this case. Rabbi Moshe Tendler writes:

> Some patients enter the consulting room saying, as the Bible records Rachel saying to Jacob, "Give me children or else I will die." [Here the benefits certainly are larger than the risks.] If a woman is toying with the idea of in vitro fertilization but is also considering going to an adoption agency, and can't make up her mind, then the physician should encourage her to recognize the risks involved and not undertake the procedure. . . . There are obstetricians and gynecologists who do not hesitate to recommend pregnancy to a woman for whom delivery means a caesarean section. . . . When there is no chance of natural delivery, with its lesser risks, physicians do subject the woman to anesthesia and to caesarean section. The risk has been accepted by our society. . . . When compared to the currently accepted standard of ethics, the risks of in vitro fertilization are no more unusual than may be incurred in the normal management of obstetric–gynecologic problems.[53]

b. Fetal risk factors. Two factors must be evaluated. Maternal risk for maternal benefit is acceptable. But fetal risk for maternal benefit poses a serious ethical problem. An axiom of

52. *Compendium*, p. 50.
53. Moshe D. Tendler, "Rabbinic Comment: In Vitro Fertilization and Extrauterine Pregnancy ('Test-Tube' Baby)" *Mount Sinai Journal of Medicine*, Vol. 51 No. 1 (Jan-Feb. 1984), p. 8.

Jewish ethics is that man is not in man's service. How can we subject the fetus to risk of injury or abnormality for parental benefit? We can, because animal studies indicate that in vitro fertilization poses negligible fetal risk. The scientific assumption is that similar low risk applies to the human fetus. The advantage of being born to parents desirous of raising a family outweighs the possible risk of abnormality.

What is the status of the fertilized egg with respect to "humanhood"? The Vatican's *Instruction* considers life as begun from the moment of fertilization. Judaism considers the fertilized egg to be potential life, but not yet actual life. Upon ethical analysis, can we equate the fertilized egg in a test tube in the two-cell stage, or the four-cell stage, or the eight-cell stage with the same egg implanted in the uterus? Judaism's answer is that there is no comparison.

Rabbi Tendler states: "Is it not a fair analysis to say that until the egg has been placed in a natural environment in which it can achieve its full potential, it should not be equated with an early abortion?"[54] Therefore a fertilized egg, not in the womb but in the environment of a test tube in which it can never attain viability, does not yet have humanhood. It may be discarded or used for the advancement of scientific knowledge.

Surrogate, Host, or Incubator Mothers

The implantation of a fertilized egg in a host womb to overcome the infertility of both parents raises the issue of maternal parenthood as well as that of donor insemination (A.I.D.).[55] In such cases the donor of the sperm is surely the father, but motherhood of such a conceptus is in question. Fatherhood is determined genetically, because the male contribution is limited to the genes carried by the sperm. But

---

54. Tendler, loc. cit., p. 9.
55. Ibid.

motherhood is both genetic (nature) and gestational (nurture). The genetic nature of the ovum is that of the donor mother, but its gestational influences are those of the surrogate, or incubator, mother.[56]

These procedures are permissible only in the absence of an alternative. They may not be resorted to by fertile parents who prefer the services of an incubator mother. This destroys the natural family bond for convenience, with unknown psychological and spiritual consequences. It poses the risk of inviting improper commerce in babies, donor organs, and the like.[57] Nevertheless, in the event that fertility cannot be otherwise attained, some authorities maintain that it is permitted in Jewish law to resort to these techniques. There is no objection on the grounds that they contravene nature or the natural conjugal act. Judaism stresses the use and judicial management of nature for attainment of the great goal of overcoming the illness of sterility. Those who forbid such techniques do so because of where they might lead, because of the inability to control the motivation of such arrangements, and especially because of the problem of enslavement of one person, using his or her body for the benefit of another person.

Embryo Transfer

In vivo fertilization, or "adoptive pregnancy," is a non-surgical alternative for a situation of non-functioning ovaries rather than blocked tubes. A woman donor is artificially inseminated and, within the first week of pregnancy, the resulting embryo is flushed from her womb and transferred to the womb of another woman who will carry it to term and be known as the baby's mother. This poses halakhic problems in that both genetic and gestational characteristics of the first mother may

---

56. *Compendium*, pp. 50–51.
57. Ibid., pp. 50–51.

be sufficient to grant her actual maternity. There is Rabbinic discussion and disagreement regarding which is, according to Jewish law, considered the mother; the host mother by whose nurture the baby is brought to term, or the biological mother who donated the egg that determines the genetic composition of the offspring.[58] Rabbi M. Feinstein suggests that though the majority opinion holds the host mother to be the parent, one must also take into account the maternal relationship of the biological mother. Jewish law would then accept both relationships, ruling strictly in each case. For instance; sexual relations with a sibling from either mother would be considered possible incest. This is not the case in testicular transplants where the sperm produced is considered by halakhah as belonging exclusively to the host. While it is true that in all other cases of transplant surgery the body part belongs to the host, the case of a woman having donated an egg as well as the case of an ovarian transplant would be different, both having a halakhic claim to parenthood. Dr. Rosner points out the biological difference between an ovarian transplant and testicular transplant, explaining that in the case of a testicular transplant, the sperm are to be produced in the future. The ovary, however, already contains the primordial egg cells at the time of the transplant. Though the gamete maintains its own individuality and retains the genetic code of the donor without reflecting the genetic code of the recipient, the fact remains that the sperm is manufactured by the host, while the eggs were already present at the time of transplant.[59] It would therefore be consistent to say that testicular transplants become part of the host, while egg donations as well as ovarian trasplants are more ambiguous, retaining more of the "maternity" of the donor.

---

58. J. David Bleich, *Judaism and Healing*, "Host Mothers," p. 93.
59. Fred Rosner, *Modern Medicine and Jewish Ethics*, (Ktav Publishing House, New Jersey, 1986), pp. 122f.

Ongoing Discussion

The question of whether surrogate motherhood violates morality and *halakhah* is actually still in dispute. Rabbi Jakobovits (19) maintains that surrogacy should never be permitted. He writes: "All forms of 'Surrogate Mothers,' 'Womb-Leasing' and 'Egg-Donation' are morally and socially repugnant as a violation of human dignity, a breach of the marriage bond, and an infringement of the inalienable rights of children."[60]

Nevertheless, the Medical Ethics Committee of the Federation considers that there are some situations where surrogacy could be condoned. Rabbi Tendler's comment expresses this view: "Clearly, if there ever were a situation in which a woman wanted to incubate an egg as an act of kindness to allow the woman who otherwise couldn't possibly conceive have the experience of motherhood, the act would be a charitable act."[61]

It is therefore obvious that the use of host or surrogate mothers for the convenience of couples able to conceive cannot be condoned. A sterile couple, however, may have recourse to a surrogate mother in the absence of alternatives, to effect pregnancy and thus save a marriage or bring happiness to the depressed. They may do so only within the limits of halakhah. There should, of course, also be absolute assurance that the surrogate is participating without coercion and with fully informed consent, and that the arrangement is protected by all necessary legal and social safeguards.[62]

Fetal Medicine

Recently, with the growth of interest in fetal tissue for a wide variety of experimentation and experimental treatment (such

---

60. I. Jakobovits, *Submission to the Warnock Committee of Inquiry*, p. 10.
61. Moshe D. Tendler, "Rabbinic Comment, In Vitro Fertilization," *The Mount Sinai Journal of Medicine*, p. 9.
62. *Compendium*, p. 52.

as for Alzheimer's disease) the issue of use of fetal tissue as well as its creation has come to the fore.

a. Research. The fetus, when out of the uterus, must be granted full protection from any damage or risk. Non-viability of fetuses is to be viewed as a fatal illness, prohibiting any active intervention to hasten death. The benefits to be accrued from such research must be relinquished in favor of the sanctity of life, even transient life.

b. Use of fetal tissue: There is medical controversy about whether fetal tissue is less likely to be rejected after transplantation. One school holds that there is no immunological benefit from fetal tissue over tissue from any other source.[63] Another group of researchers hold that fetal tissue transplants are so successful that they may raise the possibility of treatment for Parkinson's disease and other chronic illnesses.[64] If this is proven, it would make fetal tissue particularly valuable for transplantation surgery and other life-giving uses. Whereas the fetus is to be protected from risk due to research, the use of fetal tissue from a fetus that was never viable or is no longer alive would surely be permissible. The definition of death should be strictly observed according to standard halakhic criteria. Parents should be encouraged to find some solace in the life-giving contribution of the aborted fetus.[65]

Limiting use of the fetus for research to the first fourteen days is arbitrary. So what if the placenta can be perceived? We are more concerned with the motivation for the creation of

---

63. Tuch B. E., Sheil A.G.R., "Long Term Survival of Human Fetal Pancreatic Tissue Transplanted . . ." *Diabetic Medicine* 1986; 3: 24-28. Hayward A.R. and Ezer. G., "Development of Lymphocyte Populations in the Human Fetal Thymus and Spleen," *Clin. Exp. Immunol.* 1974); 17: 169-178.
64. Mahowald, Silver and Ratcheson, "The Ethical Options in Transplanting Fetal Tissue," *The Hastings Center Report* (February 1987), pp. 9–15 and references.
65. *Compendium*, pp. 52–54.

the embryo. We are concerned that embryos shall not be created for the purpose of research. We are also concerned about the use of tissue for medical purposes from stillborn babies, from aborted babies that may still be alive, and from fetuses that are not viable. If the tissue is to be used for the sake of saving life, the same criteria that apply to viable humans must apply here. Is it alive? Then it may not be used. Does it meet the criteria of death? Then it may be used.

Question: (From the Human Fertilization and Embryology Authority. They had issued a study paper on various areas of sex selection, fetal medicine, fetal research, tissue donation, and egg donation. The full and official answer was given by the Chief Rabbi and the Chief Rabbi Emeritus. The following comments address certain issues included in their answer.) Under what conditions will Judaism permit the use of fetal tissue and of eggs harvested from fetuses? Will Judaism permit use of zygotes to allow posthumous children to be born?

Answer: Judaism does not prohibit the use of fetuses and fetal material to save life. There is no difference in this respect between tissue donation from the dead and non-vital tissue donation from the living. But there is a very serious difference in that every possible safeguard must be maintained to insure that the source of fetal tissue be limited to "spares," so that abortions not be performed for the sake of harvesting tissue. It must also be ascertained that the fetus meets all the accepted criteria of human death before using its tissue.

Use of eggs harvested from fetuses is an entirely different, and in our view an even more serious matter. We do not regard legal arrangements as able in any way to supersede or override biology. Since many eggs can be harvested from one ovary (not quite a million at birth), there is serious danger of several babies being born who are biologically half brothers or half sisters. Since the source of the eggs is not recorded, there is a real possibility of consanguineous marriages, considered incestuous in Judaism's view. We are, therefore, gravely concerned about this issue.

Posthumous children are a social and psychological concern, but not a halakhic concern for Judaism. We care, but cannot say it is prohibited. The issue of consanguinity, on the other hand, is far more serious and should by itself prohibit the harvesting of eggs from such a source.

Artificial Insemination by Donor

Question: Your letter, declaring that Artificial Insemination by Donor (A.I.D.) is forbidden to Jews, distresses Jewish families as well as non-Jewish families who are suffering the agony of infertility. By referring to parenthood as a blessing, you imply that infertility is a punishment. Would it not have been better to say forthrightly say that A.I.D. is forbidden in order not to thwart God's will that such couples remain infertile?

Answer: The letter that provoked the above comment was only partially printed in the London *Times* on January 17, 1994, as follows:

> Judaism has long wrestled with issues that relate to the use of fetal eggs and ovarian tissue for implantation and transplant. Recognizing parenthood as a blessing and humanity as God's partner in the work of creation, it welcomes medical advances in the treatment of fertility.
>
> But there must be limits if our most fundamental values are not to be put at risk. Childhood is set in the ethical con-

text of the family, the sacred bond uniting personal identity, love, and nurturing.

For that reason, while Judaism is generally sympathetic to treatments which allow an otherwise infertile couple to conceive, it is opposed to the use of donated sperm or ova. This breaks the genetic connection between parents and child and introduces confusion at the most basic level of identity and relationship. May we bring a child into the world who can say "I am" and cannot answer the question "Who am I?" It is this, rather than the age of the host mother or the color of the baby's skin, that is the central ethical question to be addressed.

Since the newspaper severely edited the original letter, what emerged could easily be misunderstood. I believe that is why you are so concerned. Here are the points in the original letter that were omitted:

The principles Judaism applies to such questions include the following:

1. Man has a task on earth to use nature for his benefit, and in the process of innovation, invention, and discovery, he becomes a partner with God in creation.
2. The duty to procreate is the first imperative of the Bible (Gen. 1:28; 9:1).
3. The duty to preserve human life and health is a religious duty (Deut. 4:9, 15) which includes the Divine permission to intervene in the course of nature when necessary (Ex. 21:19).
4. Judaism treats infertility as an illness to be overcome by means of the scientist's skill.

But there are limits.

1. Judaism forbids abortion, except for grave physical or psychological hazard to the health of the mother.
2. The family is a sacred unit to be enhanced and preserved. Insemination of single women is opposed.

3. Judaism's has a strict code of sex and morality and absolutely prohibits incest (Deut. 4:9,15).
4. To Judaism, biological facts cannot be overturned by laws or by society's usage. Genetic relationships cannot be denied or overridden by legislation.

Judaism will therefore condone and encourage methods to increase the possibility of birth for otherwise barren women. It would oppose any practice which would prevent the certain establishment of genetic identity, for this creates the possibility of sibling incestuous marriage. A fetus is born with more than a million eggs. There is a strong possibility that many women might be implanted with eggs from the same fetus. Judaism would oppose this, for it can lead to sibling marriages. This is one of the reasons Judaism ordinarily opposes artificial insemination by a donor other than the husband.

Many complex questions in this area are being discussed by Rabbis, such as: who owns the fetus? May we use its tissue for non-life-threatening illness such as we deem infertility to be? Judaism will not be troubled by the age of the mother. After all, Sarah was 100 when she bore Isaac. Nor will it be concerned about skin pigmentation. It is, however, definitely concerned about "designer babies" and sees dire consequences for society at the bottom of that slope.

It is little wonder, then, that you misunderstood the intent of my letter. To be specific:

Parenthood is indeed a blessing. But infertility is not a punishment. It is a tragedy and should be overcome as best we can. This does not mean that we may achieve such a goal through improper means. One of the serious problems of donated sperm or ova is consanguinity. You will note that from one fetus over a million eggs can be recovered. Even if a half dozen are fertilized from such eggs, they are in fact biological half brothers or sisters.

Laws in England require that we keep no records of who the donors are. This means that it could become very easy for biological brothers and sisters to marry each other. This has indeed happened in other parts of the world. What I have described to you is the main objection to donor eggs or sperm in a country like ours that does not allow records to be kept of the biological father or mother. There are, however, other reasons too. Suffice it to say that each case has to be dealt with separately, on its own merits.

On the other hand, Judaism is very strongly in favor of adoption, maintaining that those who raise someone else's child in their own home practices charity every moment of every day. If in vitro fertilization cannot help, adoption might. I know how difficult adoption is. But it is possible, and when all else fails, we believe it is certainly preferable to doing something that Jewish law forbids.

Finally, although most Jewish authorities do not condone the use of donor sperm for artificial insemination (A.I.D.), the vast majority maintain that those who have nevertheless used this method carry no stigma of adultery, nor do the offspring who are produced bear any stigma of bastardy in Jewish law.

Embryo Research

Questions: I am currently researching for a piece of work that contributes towards an MSc in Psychology and Health at Middlesex University. My first joint degree was in Genetics and Cell Biology with Science and Society at Manchester University. I have become increasingly interested and concerned about developments in biotechnology. The theme of the essay is the moral status of the embryo, given the imperatives of IVF that create excess embryos. I am seeking to deal with the issue of when life begins and the uses to which spare embryos can be put. I would therefore particularly appreciate receiving a Jewish perspective on IVF possibilities and problems and on the moral status of the embryo according to Judaism.

(On the same subject, from Australia): I am the Fertility Center Counselor at Lingard Fertility Clinic, and this clinic is presently considering the ethics of embryo donation with a view to deciding whether to implement such a program. Concurrently, I have also undertaken a University Masters' project entitled "Embryo Donation—the Ethico-Legal Issues and a Process Protocol." I hope to identify the issues and then design a preliminary donation protocol that addresses these issues. So I am writing to you to seek from you the Jewish viewpoint on embryo donation. I realize that there may be a spectrum of ideas and concerns within Judaism.

Answer: Lord Jakobovits, in his submission to the Warnock Committee and in his address to the House of Lords, wrote and spoke on the status of the embryo and experimentation on it. Following are excerpts from his address and his report:

> I do not accept that full human status necessarily starts at conception though I have a profound respect for that view. Nor do I want to see an absolute ban on all embryo experiments.
>
> These are my principal concerns. It is surely repugnant to generate human life solely for the purpose of destroying it, in other words, to produce embryos only to destroy them by experiments. However diverse our views on the exact moment when the embryo begins to enjoy full human status, no one can deny that so long as it has a potential for human life its status is no longer that of a mere egg or mere sperm. An embryo which can develop into a human being must really be entitled to supreme respect and protection. At the same time one must recognise that those who support certain experiments are equally concerned to promote human life by eliminating the afflictions of infertility and of grave genetic defects which often lead to premature death.
>
> Are these two concerns really incompatible? I believe that they can easily be reconciled in a simple and yet effective formula.

The proposed amendments seek first to ensure that no human embryo should ever be generated solely for the purpose of research. The potential of human life must never be used simply as a means in this way.

Secondly, they seek to restrict research to such embryos as had to be produced to bring about a live birth. There is then no reason why an excess embryo should not be used in that way, once it becomes impossible for it to develop into a live baby.

Thirdly, the research to be done on these so-called 'spare' embryos should be strictly limited to vital therapeutic purpose; namely, the relief of infertility and the prevention of the transmission of grave genetic abnormalities.[66]

The same point was made by Lord Jakobovits in his 1984 submission to the Warnock Committee of Inquiry on the Jewish view of Human Fertilization and Embryology:

There are serious objections, based on the mechanization of human procreation and the consequent degradation of all human life, to the generation of human embryos purely for experimental use or for organ transplant purposes. Any technique which involves breeding whole embryos for the sake of the desired organ, the rest of the genetic material to be discarded afterwards, would reduce the creation of life to the manufacture of supplies for laboratories and assembly lines for ersatz organs.

But eggs originally fertilized for re-implantation into the mother (in excess of the number actually so used) may serve for experimentation so long as they could still be used as "spares" to achieve a successful pregnancy. Thereafter they should be discarded without delay.[67]

---

66. I. Jakobovits, *House of Lords Official Report Parliamentary Debates, Hansard*, (London, Tuesday, March 6, 1990), Vol. 516 No. 50, pp. 1059f.

67. I. Jakobovits, "Human Fertilisation and Embryology, a Jewish View," *Submissions to the Warnock Committee of Inquiry and*

Lord Jakobovits explained Judaism's view of the treatment of handicapped newborns as follows:

A physically or mentally abnormal child has the same claim to life as a normal child because it is considered a person (*nefesh*).

Furthermore, while only the killing of a born and viable child constitutes murder in Jewish law, the destruction of the fetus, too, is a moral offense and cannot be justified except out of consideration for the mother's life or health. Consequently, the fear that a child may or will be deformed is not in itself a legitimate indication for its abortion, particularly since there is usually a chance that the child might turn out to be quite normal. Killing a handicapped adult is similarly prohibited.[68]

There is important material in the *Compendium of Jewish Medical Ethics* as follows:

Surgical intervention to prevent death of the fetus should be contemplated even if, on a neonate, the risk would have precluded such surgery. The certainty of a still-birth is not to be compared to the certainty of fatal outcome for a pediatric patient. A fetus in the process of maturation has not yet attained full viability. The high-risk surgery does not impugn its status of potential life, but is a result of it. Whereas abortion of a viable fetus is the "killing of potential life," the attempt to give life to an ill fetus is justified by possible benefit rather than risks involved.

Fetal Research: The large number of medically supervised abortions has made available fetal organs and tissues, as well as the immature fetus itself, for developmental, immunological, and other studies. The fetus, when out of the uterus, must

---

the Department of Health and Social Security, by the Chief Sir Immanuel Jakobovits, (Office of the Chief Rabbi, London, 1984), p. 9.

68. I. Jakobovits, in *The Jewish Review*, London, Nov. 14, 1962.

be granted full protection from any damage or risk. The non-viability of these fetuses is to be viewed as a fatal illness, proscribing any active intervention to hasten death. The benefits to be accrued from such research must be relinquished in favor of the sanctity of life—even transient life.

Immunological studies indicate that fetal tissues have reduced antigenicity. This makes them particularly valuable for transplantation surgery. Whereas the fetus is to be protected from risk due to research, the use of fetal tissue after the fetus is no longer alive, as defined by neurological or cardiopulmonary criteria, is surely permissible. Parents should be encouraged to find some solace in the life-giving contribution of the aborted fetus.

Whereas "banking" of tissues from adult autopsies cannot be approved, tissue from non-viable fetuses (after expiration) may be banked for future use or subsequent burial.[69]

Additional sources for your research might include the chapter on "Ethics of Reproductive Medicine" in the 1993 *Jews' College Centre for Medical Ethics Yearbook*[70] and Dr. Fred Rosner's *Modern Medicine and Jewish Ethics*.[71] These sources will give you an overview of this area, and in the notes you will find many more sources for additional research. Finally, an article by me which includes material on this subject appeared in the Australia and *New Zealand Jewish Year Book*, 1988.[72]

---

69. *Compendium on [Jewish] Medical Ethics* (Federation of Jewish Philanthropies of New York, Sixth Edition, 1984), pp. 53f.
70. Professor Robert Winston and Dayan Ivan Binstock, "Ethics of Reproductive Medicine," *Yearbook of the Centre for Medical Ethics, Jews' College*, Vol. I, (London, 1993), available through Jews' College, 44a Albert Road, Hendon NW4.
71. Ktav Publishing House Inc. (Hoboken, New Jersey) and Yeshiva University Press, (New York 1986).
72. Ed. Jacqueline Langley (Abbotsford, Victoria 1988), pp. 82–88.

Circumcision

Question (From Dr. Bernard Tuch, University of Sydney Department of Medicine): We would like to use foreskins for research and experimental treatment. The custom in Judaism is to bury them. Would this be fulfilled by covering a closed container in which they are kept with sterile sand and then washing it off?

Answer: I had a chance to discuss the matter with the head of the Beth Din, Dayan Ehrentrau, and also with the Chief Rabbi, although very briefly. The following answer has their mutual concurrence.

Covering a container in which the foreskins are placed will not do. The preferable method is to use sterile sand, if possible, to cover them and then wash them off. If this will not be acceptable, then use the foreskins without covering them with anything. But be sure to take any residue that remains after use for your research and bury it. Thus, if there are any foreskins or parts of foreskins remaining, they must be buried after you are through with them.

Rabbi Moshe Dovid Tendler disagrees. He notes that foreskins are now used in life-saving therapy. The custom of burying foreskins does not have halakhic import. It would therefore be permitted to use foreskins for the purpose indicated.[73]

Question (From Jeremy Jones, Executive Vice President, Executive Council of Australian Jewry): The Law Reform Commission of the State of Queensland has commenced an inquiry

---

73. Moshe Dovid Tendler in a private communication with me.

into the circumcision of male children, on the extraordinary basis that the operation is performed without the consent of the child. While we have collected a great deal of argumentation from Australian sources, I would be grateful if you could urgently forward to this office any good material which could be sent on in original or amended form to the Queensland Law Reform Commission.

Answer: It is totally illogical for them to argue that circumcision be forbidden on an infant since consent cannot be obtained, and to blithely permit all sorts of other operations, even cosmetic ones, simply by the request of the parents or with their consent, since they are indeed proper surrogates in this matter. Nevertheless, since you are dealing with a public effort that has emotional overtones, and since there may be some in the camp of the advocates of the proposed measure who have motives far from altruistic, it is important that you be equipped with as much documentary evidence as possible. So I am sending you some material about circumcision that you can use. This includes:

1. A statement from Donald Gribetz, M. D. Dr. Gribetz is one of the foremost pediatricians in the United States, a Professor of Pediatrics at the Mount Sinai Medical Center. He is also very active in the Commission on Medical Ethics, Federation of Jewish Philanthropies, New York, and I have taken it upon myself to forward the Queensland request to him since he has a great deal of material at hand regarding circumcision. He writes:

> *Brith milah*, or ritual circumcision, is a fundamental tenet of Jewish tradition. "God further said to Abraham: 'As for you, you shall keep my covenant, you and your offspring to come throughout the ages. Such shall be the covenant which you shall keep, between Me and you and your offspring to follow: every male among you shall be circumcised. You shall circumcise the flesh of your foreskin· and that shall be the sign of

the covenant between Me and you. At the age of eight days every male among you throughout the generations shall be circumcised'" (Gen. 17:9–12). It was re-emphasized when God spoke to Moses: "When a woman at childbirth bears a male . . . on the eighth day the flesh of his foreskin shall be circumcised" (Lev. 12:1–3).

Ritual circumcision of males has been practiced by Jews for thousands of years in accordance with the above biblical commandments. Circumcision in the Jewish tradition has not been performed for any primary surgical or medical indications. Nevertheless, it is our responsibility to reconcile the ritual procedure with up-to-date medical thinking.

With the adverse publicity that circumcision as a surgical procedure has been receiving, it is of great interest that several recent studies have suggested an advantageous medical outcome of this procedure. Evidence is accumulating that urinary tract infections in circumcised males are less frequent than in non-circumcised males. In fact, the American Academy of Pediatrics has formed a task force to evaluate these data.

Another aspect of circumcision is the question of pain experienced by the infant. Several groups are investigating different methods of analgesia. If a feasible method is devised, there is no objection in Jewish tradition to incorporation.

Dr. Gribetz cited a number of studies, included the sources, and I forwarded the following material to be included:

1. The most recent report of the Task Force on circumcision of the American Academy of Pediatrics. This is an official reversal of two previous reports, due largely to recent studies which show less urinary tract infections in circumcised males.[74]

---

74. Dr. Edgar J. Schoen, "The Status of Circumcision of Newborns," *The New England Journal of Medicine*, May 3, 1990, Vol. 322, No. 18, pp. 1308ff, and the "Report of the Task Force on Circumcision, American Academy of Pediatrics, *Pediatrics*, August 1989, Vol. 84 No. 4, pp. 388ff.

2. Two representative articles by Dr. Wiswell concerning the decreased incidence of urinary tract infections in circumcised males. Wiswell was the original "discoverer" and publicist of this problem; his studies have been corroborated by others.[75]

3. A recent article concerning attempts to alleviate pain in circumcision. If successful this will answer some of the critics of the procedure. In addition, nowhere is it stated that brith must be painful.[76]

4. Two articles summarizing the data which are accumulating to emphasize the benefits of circumcision. Dr. Schoen's statements are in two prestigious journals, *New England Journal of Medicine* and *Pediatrics*.[77]

Dr. Gribetz concludes his letter as follows:

Finally, neither I nor any one consulted ever have heard of the preposterous suggestion that a neonate should by himself give consent for the procedure. One day or one week infants frequently require emergency cardiac or gastrointestinal surgery. They do not give consent; their parents do.

I also included the following information in the "package":

---

75. Major Thomas E. Wiswell MC USA, LTCol Franklin R. Smith MC USA, Col James W. Bass MC USA, "Decreased Incidence of Urinary Tract Infections in Circumcised Male Infants," *Pediatrics*, May 1985, Vol. 75 No. 5, pp. 90ff; and LTC Thomas E. Wiswell MC USA and Col Dietrich W. Geschke MC USA (from Medical Research Fellowship, Walter Reed Army Institute of Research, Wash. D.C.), "Risks From Circumcision During the First Month of Life Compared with those for Uncircumcised Boys," Pediatrics, June 1989, Vol. 83 No. 6, pp. 1011ff.

76. Weatherstone, Rasmussen, Erenberg, Jackson, Claflin and Leff, "Safety and Efficacy of a Topical Anesthetic for Neonatal Circumcision," *Pediatrics*, November 1993, Vol. 92 No. 5, pp. 710ff.

77. Edgar J. Schoen MD, Kaiser Permanente Medical Center, Oakland CA., "The Status of Circumcision of Newborns," *The New England Journal of Medicine*, May 3, 1990, Vol. 322 No. 18, pp. 1308ff., and Schoen "Circumcision Updated - Indicated?," *Pediatrics*, Sept. 1993, pp. 860ff.

1. A memo from the Brith Milah Board of New York, Inc., which addresses the use of EMLA, a topical anesthetic, for milah, and reports that rabbis have approved of use of EMLA for this purpose.[78]

I also relayed to Australia a great deal of additional information received from New York concerning circumcision which they subsequently used with success. The inquiry was eventually dropped, only to be renewed several years later.

Subsequently, a responsum by Rabbi Dr. Moshe Dovid Tendler on the issue of EMLA for circumcision appeared, in which he stated that it is not only permitted but required by Jewish law. For if it eliminates or mitigates pain, we must use it, since we are forbidden to cause unnecessary pain to any human being.[79] Still later, Rabbi Tendler concluded that authoritative studies had been made that indicate that topical anesthetic is safe and effective and should be used. He has also indicated that 30% lidocaine is even more effective than EMLA and should be the anesthetic of choice.[80]

In the course of this correspondence, I received a letter from Dr. David A. Blackman of Ottawa, Ontario, an Anglican priest, who writes as follows:

---

78. A research project was reported in *The Journal of the American Medical Association* (JAMA, August 18, 1993), Vol 270 No. 7, pp. 850ff., that a topical anaesthetic can be used effectively to eliminate pain during a circumcision. The anesthetic cream is EMLA and it has been used in Europe. . . . The Brith Milah Board of New York recommends that this cream be used, after consulting with the baby's pediatrician.

79. Moshe D. Tendler, halakhic decisor of the Board, ruled that since . . . a small sample size . . . were circumcised in this . . . trial, its use can not yet be made mandatory. After numerous children are anesthetized with EMLA, it will be incumbent on Mohelim to use this cream and thus avoid causing needless pain, based on "He shall not cause suffering" (Deut. 25:3 as cited in Talmud Makkot 23a).

80. See Weatherstone, Rasmussen et all, "Safety and Efficacy of a Topical Anesthetic for Neonatal Circumcision," *Pediatrics* 1993, 92:710–714.

I thought you would find the enclosed of interest, and I sincerely hope that you will be as concerned about this as I am. Over the past twenty to twenty-five years, anti-circumcisionists in North America have greatly contributed to the myths, prejudices (personal and religious), and ignorance that still surround the issue of circumcision. These people do not respect other people's rights, opinions, or beliefs, as long as their point of view is [considered] the only acceptable one. The publicity campaign that the NO-CIRC organization instigated in 1987 regarding the circumcised or uncircumcised status of the sons of the Prince and Princess of Wales is a perfect example of what anti-circumcisionists will do in order to gain converts to their cause.

Although I am not Jewish but Anglican by faith, I believe in the preventive health measures that circumcision accords our male population. Based on my research, I consider the non-Jewish populations to be poorly educated on this health issue. To this end, I have been actively involved in trying to encourage our medical profession to provide unbiased and informative educational material to the general public. Whenever I can, I publicly challenge misleading views being expressed by "antis" in newspaper and magazine articles.

The responses I have received from many in the medical profession have been most favorable, and I feel my efforts have not been in vain. I was much encouraged when I received public recognition of my efforts and support from Dr. A. J. Fink (a urologist residing in California) in his book entitled *Circumcision—a Parent's Decision for Life.*

When one sees articles written by "antis" maintaining that circumcision causes crib deaths and divorce, that all circumcised males are neurotic, rapists, or homosexuals, that circumcised males are more accident-prone and self-destructive and more prone to violent and non-violent suicides, it is very clear just how regressive their campaign really is.

Since 1987 the "antis" in North America, through a group called NO-CIRC, have received a great deal of unwarranted publicity at the expense of the sons of the Prince and Princess of Wales. They issued a press release that year naming the Prince and Princess of Wales "Parents of the Year" because, supposedly, the royal couple did not have their sons circumcised.

NO-CIRC obtained their hearsay information from a "Cut/Uncut" celebrity list originating from California. The author of this list obtained his information from a tabloid called *The National Inquirer.*

NO-CIRC then wrote to the Palace and the Palace would not confirm the information that NO-CIRC presented. This was brought to light in an article that appeared in *FQ*, which is published by a group that call themselves "Uncircumcised Society of America."

I am not one to accept hearsay information, so I have been conducting my own investigation on this matter. I first wrote to one of the medical advisors to the British royal family. I informed him that anti-circumcisionists and the tabloid trade were maintaining that the Princess of Wales refused to have her sons circumcised.

The reply I received from the medical advisor stated, "In my opinion, without seeing the tabloids, the information that they have is purely speculative."

I then wrote to the Assistant Secretary to the Princess of Wales and informed her that various writers of books and magazines were maintaining that the princess had made statements against circumcision. I have enclosed a reply that I received from the Palace on the matter I raised, [to the effect that the Princess never made a public statement on the issue].

Question: I subsequently received a query from Suzanne F. Singer, Managing Editor, *Moment Magazine*, Washington DC, who asked about the circumcision of the children of the British royal family. She had heard that they used a *mohel* for that purpose and asked me to corroborate or deny this on the basis of my local knowledge.

Answer: I too have heard the anecdotal report that they have used a *mohel.*

I made some investigations and came up with "good news and bad news." Dr. Sifman, the medical officer of the Initiation Society, the Chief Rabbi's organization for supervision of *mohelim,* assures me that the Prince of Wales, Prince Charles, was indeed circumcised by a mohel, the late Dr. Snowman, who was a medical man as well. It is an old royal family tradition that they be circumcised. A Jewish *mohel* had been chosen, probably following a tradition that dates at least from the time of Queen Victoria.

There were two possible reasons for such a choice. First, the *mohel* was considered to have better experience in the technique of the operation. Second, Queen Victoria was under the impression that the royal family of Britain was descendent from ancient Israel, and possibly from the family of King David. In fact, it had long been the custom to call the first-born son of the royal family David. Thus King Edward the Eighth, who had abdicated, possessed the name David amongst his other first names and titles, and in the intimate circle of the family was actually called David.

That was the good news. The bad news is that the detractors of circumcision among the practitioners of medicine convinced the Prince and Princess of Wales to dispense with circumcision. That is why the new generation of royalty is uncircumcised.

Sex Selection

Question: A number of questions have been asked about the claims that sex selection of infants is now possible. Some have come from students, such as the following:

"Recently, an organization called the London Clinic has claimed to have in use a system whereby, on payment of a fee, prospective parents can be guided and instructed about how they can choose the sex of a child yet to be born to them. A high rate of success is claimed. In my dissertation I should like to include information from the leaders of the three major religions in this country on the subject."

Another query came from Professor Colin Campbell, Chairman of the The Human Fertilization and Embryology Authority. They had issued a consultation document on the subject and have asked for comments.

Answer: Following is a summary of the approach Judaism takes to gender selection.

It would be permitted to select sex for disease-related reasons provided this was done within certain limits. One of the limits is to avoid abortion. Thus sex selection after natural fertilization takes place, by checking the sex of the embryo and aborting the unwanted one, is absolutely forbidden, for abortion is permitted only when the life of the mother is threatened.[81]

Sex predetermination and selection may be regarded with more leniency if it is done before implantation, such as in a procedure of in vitro fertilization, where a number of harvested eggs from the mother are fertilized by the husband's sperm and two or more are selected for implantation. It is permitted, at this stage, to select non-disease-carrying fertilized eggs for implantation. In an attempt to avoid genetic transfer of sex-related diseases, it may be impossible to determine

---

81. J. D. Bleich, "Abortion in Halakhic Literature," in *Contemporary Halachic Problems* (New York: Ktav and Yeshiva University Press, 1977), pp. 325–371; D. M. Feldman, *Marital Relations, Birth Control, and Abortion in Jewish Law* (New York: Schocken, 1975), pp. 251–294; I. Jakobovits, "Jewish Views on Abortion," in *Jewish Bioethics*, ed. F. Rosner and J.D. Bleich (New York, Hebrew Publishing Company, 1979), pp. 118–133.

which are potential carriers except by choosing the sex that does not carry the disease. In such a case it would be appropriate to choose the disease-free sex for implantation, since this is done for therapeutic reasons.

The requirement of Judaism that the commandment to be fruitful and multiply is not satisfied until at least a boy and a girl are produced should not lead to sex selection. The spirit of the command is to propagate, and not limit propagation exclusively to two offspring. "Be fruitful and multiply" is in fact interpreted to mean that a family should continue to propagate until there is at least one child of each sex. Social reasons should not be used as an excuse for sex selection.

It is, however, possible for a woman who has had many children of one sex to feel herself threatened by continued pregnancy; or physicians may indicate that continued pregnancy beyond one more attempt might be harmful to her, and she wants to take one last chance to have a child of the other sex. Such a situation may be regarded by halakhic authorities as therapeutic in nature and sex selection might be permitted. Of course, the limitation that such selection be done before implantation, and that it should not lead to abortion, must be observed. The questions and concerns about semen collection are less severe and restrictive if the procedure has a therapeutic purpose.

There are other methods of sex selection that Rabbis of the Talmud appeared to permit. Thus, the Talmud suggests various ways to increase the chances of having male or female progeny result from intercourse.[82] All these methods have in common that there is no abortion, and that they are advice to the couple for procedures before, during, or after intercourse. From this it can be inferred that sex selection methods that depend on natural conditions, such as acidity or

---

82. Talmud *Niddah* 31a,b, 25b, and 28a; *Gittin* 57a; *Berachot* 54a. *Cf.* Rosner, *Modern Medicine and Jewish Ethics*, p. 130ff.

alkalinity of the vagina, time of intercourse after ovulation, special diets, and the like, are all permitted.

Question: I am particularly interested in the method developed by Ericcson in America whereby sperms are separated in an albumen gradient and then used to fertilize a human ovum in vitro before reintroducing it to the womb. The method is fairly accurate if a couple desires a male child. What is the view of Judaism?

Answer: In vitro fertilization and all other forms of birth assistance are therapies with attendant risk. We may submit to the risk only for cure of a condition of illness that warrants taking such a risk. We consider childlessness an illness, and its cure well worth the risk involved in the protocol required for IVF. That is not the case for sex selection.

There are certain prohibitions involved that are waived in the case of illness. For instance, masturbation is forbidden. Even when used for procreation, it is acceptable only when other methods of semen collection that Judaism would prefer, prove ineffectual. But all this would be only permitted to alleviate the stress of illness and not to fulfill a preference of sex. That is not considered therapy.

Jewish law requires that a family fulfill the commandment of procreation by having at least a boy and a girl. This is taken to mean that the family should continue to have children until that desideratum is reached. There is a terrible decrease of births in Jewish families, and the result is that we are not recreating our people. We need large families. The desired goal of large families to compensate for the drop in Jewish birth rate is negated by sex selection, which might deter families from having additional children.

Furthermore, there is a natural balance of sexes. Allowing pre-selection of sex would tend to upset this balance, especially in some communities and countries where children of a particular sex are considered more desirable.

Finally, for practical reasons we would refuse to countenance this. The entire process is very expensive and uses a great many community resources. It does not matter that the patient may have the money to spend. There is a waiting list, sometimes of years, before a vacancy occurs admitting a patient to an IVF program. Allowing someone to use the program simply for a preference of sex, or size, or genetic composition, or for any other frivolous reason might deprive a childless couple, whose needs are therapeutic, from being accepted. I have earlier indicated that from the Talmud it can be inferred that certain other forms of sex selection would be permitted. These are methods that depend on natural conditions, such as acidity or alkalinity of the vagina, time of intercourse after ovulation, special diets, and the like.

Infant Death

Question (From Reverend Ronnie Clark, Wythenshawe Hospital, University of Manchester School of Medicine): I am at present researching ways of helping families faced by the trauma of stillbirth and infant death. Can you give a guide to Jewish parents regarding stillbirth? Does Judaism have any advice to give in order to comfort families bereaved by stillbirth or infant death?

Answer: Yours is a necessary study, and a serious problem for people at a time of crisis. Ministry of presence—empathy—but no attempt to answer the questions which must arise at such a time, is the best path I can suggest. In this respect, I do not believe Judaism has any special answers to give, beyond that which humanity and common sense can provide. For at such a time Judaism does not seek to explain away the tragedy or to create a feeling of sin or guilt, but rather to simply share the burden and find a possible way for the bereaved to begin looking towards a brighter future.

The approach must differ in every situation, and not only

because the families differ in the make-up of the parents' emotional character, but also because the cases, and the conditions surrounding the stillbirth, differ too; for instance, a spontaneous abortion, whether early in term or later, a fetus or infant which perished without apparent reason, in contrast to the embryo with severe anomalies which would have precluded survival in any case, an infant which had survived less than thirty days and then died, an infant who lived for 30 days, and therefore passed the test of viability according to Jewish law, and then died.

In the same way, the feeling of hopelessness and despair of a childless family faced with the loss of their last chance for an offspring, differs from that of parents who lost a baby but who have other children.

The comfort offered to each family differs according to its personality and according to the type of tragedy it has suffered, and differs also according to the background and personality of each "comforter," be they rabbi or layman. However, neighbors (and the rabbi) must understand that to the mother a nine month baby died.

There are certain practical procedures which are to be followed when dealing with Jewish parents. The following paper, published by the Chief Rabbi's office and prepared by Rabbi Geoffrey Hyman, outlines these procedures.[83]

Rabbinical Council of the United Synagogue

Stillbirth and Neonatal Death; A Guide for the Jewish Parent
by Rabbi Geoffrey Hyman

The Jewish community would like to help you in this time of sorrow. We cannot hope, through the printed word, to alleviate your sense of grief and loss. We know, however, that the

---

83. Geoffrey Hyman "Stillbirth and Neonatal Death, A Guide For the Jewish Parent," (Office of the Chief Rabbi, London, 1992).

grief is even harder to bear when it is accompanied by uncertainty and confusion about what to do, and to whom to turn.

This leaflet is offered to clear away that uncertainty. It explains the Jewish procedures to be followed when an infant dies at birth or during the first 30 days of life.

RESPECT FOR THE BODY

A post mortem should be avoided unless there is a possibility of saving another life thereby. This includes urgent medical reasons, such as the suspicion of hereditary factors which, if ascertained, might help to save the lives of other children in the family, born or yet to be born. In the absence of such compelling reasons, a post mortem is forbidden. The respect due to a body which housed a soul applies to an infant as well. Your child possessed a pure soul; so much so, that one great sage of earlier generations instructed his family to bury him amongst the stillborn, since he had wanted to be buried amongst those who were pure.

If the hospital insists on such a procedure, or if there is doubt in your mind about the issue, please call the Jewish hospital chaplain or your rabbi who will often be able to help.

BURIAL

Burial in a Jewish cemetery is obligatory. You will need certain papers in order to receive authorization for burial. The hospital staff will be able to advise you.

To make the arrangements, contact the Burial Society through your synagogue group. If your baby is to be buried in a London United Synagogue (Orthodox) cemetery, you can initiate arrangements by phoning the United Synagogue Burial Society, (01) 387-7891, or (01) 387-4300. If they are not at the telephone, leave a message and they will call back.[84] It is

---

84. In the United States a reputable Jewish funeral home and its staff take the place of the United Synagogue Burial Society. The procedure in both countries is to contact the rabbi immediately.

advisable to inform your synagogue office of your bereavement. You should call your rabbi as soon as possible, and wherever applicable, the Jewish chaplain attached to the hospital.

THE FUNERAL SERVICE

Psalms and prayers which are usually recited at a funeral service, are appropriate (For example, Psalm 16, the Memorial Prayer and the Prayer for the Bereaved in the Singer Siddur, page 131).

There is no obligation to tear one's garments (*Kri'ah*).

The service is usually private, and a minyan is not necessary. Kaddish is also omitted.

The baby should be given a name before the funeral. A boy is nominally circumcised by the burial society when they prepare him for burial (*Tahara*), and the name is given at that time. A girl is named before the funeral service begins. We give a name in order that no Jewish life remain anonymous.

Many feel that attendance at the funeral is helpful to the bereaved, but this is entirely a matter of personal feeling. It will be understood if you do not wish to attend.

MOURNING PRACTICES

Formal mourning is not observed when an infant dies before thirty days of life. Thirty days is the period of time Jewish tradition considers necessary to determine whether the infant is definitely viable. It is required to sit *shiva* for a child who had survived beyond thirty days of life.

STONE-SETTING

A tombstone to mark the grave of your baby should be arranged. A month later is an appropriate time, though it can be delayed till later. The full name should be inscribed on the stone. Arrangements should be made through the Burial Society. They will be able to advise you if you have any question.

YAHRZEIT, THE ANNIVERSARY OF DEATH (if after 30 days of life)

You may light a Yahrzeit candle to mark the anniversary. You may also wish to attend Synagogue and to recite appropriate prayers.

4

Saving Life Through Surgery

Organ Transplants

Question (From Bill New, Senior Research Officer, King's Fund Institute): Since Orthodox groups are opposed to autopsies, how can they remove organs from cadavers for transplants? Why do you not accept brain death as the criterion of death?

Answer: Orthodox Jewish groups are not opposed to the removal of organs for transplants, since this is done in order to save life. This value of saving life takes precedence over the prohibition against deriving benefit from a corpse or disfiguring it. In fact, saving life takes precedence over all the laws of the Torah except three, the prohibition of murder, adultery, and idolatry. Thus, if we know that an organ can save a life, one should remove it for use, provided, of course, that the next of kin consents. Every effort is made by even the most pious rabbis to convince the family to permit this. (Jewish law defines "life-threatening illness" much more liberally than does the medical profession. Thus blindness is considered a life-threatening illness, since impaired sight can cause a person to fall, possibly resulting in mortal injury. Corneal transplants are therefore permitted.)

The background: there is a Biblical law requiring that even the body of an executed criminal may not be left on display overnight: "It is an abomination," for the human body, even that of a criminal who deserved the death penalty, must be respected as the repository of the soul during life. Therefore, after death, it must be buried promptly and with respect.[1]

Saving and Preserving Life

For the same reason, Jewish bereavement practices require that burial be made within a day of death. Jewish law requires that we ignore a last will or request to the effect that a person should not be buried.[2]

The next of kin is responsible for the burial. If there is no next of kin, then the entire community bears responsibility for prompt and respectful burial. This gives rise to the law that when one encounters a cadaver with no one to care for it, such as a body found in the field, one is responsible for that cadaver and may not leave it till it is buried. This even applies to those who may not otherwise become "ritually contaminated" by contact with the dead, such as priests. In fact, in olden times, while the Holy Temple stood in Jerusalem, it even applied to the High Priest on the holiest day of the year, Yom Kippur, though by caring for the cadaver he would be disqualified from officiating on behalf of all the Jewish people in the Jerusalem Temple service. For Judaism considers prompt and respectful burial to be a paramount value.[3] Nevertheless, when saving life is possible, then these values are set aside. Autopsy should take place, transplants should be made, life should be saved. More than fifty years ago, the then Sefardic Chief Rabbi of Israel, Rabbi Ben Zion Uziel, ruled as

---

1. Deuteronomy, 21:22–23, and Talmud, Sanhedrin, 46b.
2. Sanhedrin, loc. cit.
3. Leviticus 21:11, and Talmud, Sanhedrin, 47b. See also Nazir, 48b.

follows: "Anyone with a knowledge of the development and progress of medicine will not for a moment doubt the benefits that accrue from autopsies and dissections. Autopsies are of inestimable value in establishing the cause of the ailment and its effect upon other organs of the body. Where the preservation of life of the living is concerned, there is no prohibition of *nivul hames*, desecration of the body."[4]

The consensus of rabbinical opinion is, however, that the life to be saved must be before us, here and now. Otherwise, autopsy would be forbidden.[5] With modern ease of communication, many more patients with life-threatening illness can be treated by transplants from cadavers, even when far removed from the patient's location. Swift air transportation can fly a life-saving organ anywhere in the world. Jewish law takes this into account when permitting organ removal from a cadaver and considers such patients to be before us here and now because of their accessibility.

As for acceptance of brain-death criteria: we are universally opposed to using a flat encephalograph as a criterion of death. But there is an authoritative school of Jewish rabbinic opinion that accepts brain-stem death, complete cessation of blood flow to the brain, as a valid criterion of death.[6]

Question (From Mr. John M. Johnstone, Head of Religious Education at the John Warner School, Hoddenston,

---

4. Ben Tziyon Meir Hai Uziel, *Piske Uziel*, No. 30, pp. 172ff.
5. Yehezkel Landau, Responsa *Noda BiYehuda*, pt. 2, "Yoreh Deah," No. 210. See F. Rosner, *Modern Medicine and Jewish Ethics* (Ktav Publishing, Hoboken, New Jersey 1986), p. 295, nn. 4–7, for a comprehensive listing of subsequent responsa on the issue of autopsy.
6. For a complete discussion of this issue, see infra, pp. 143–145, N. E. Shulman response to Mr. Brian Glenville, reprint from the *Yearbook of the Centre for Medical Ethics*, Jews College, London, 1993, pp. 101–117.

Herts.): I am currently following up a visit by a heart transplant patient. I am trying to gather as much information as possible which deals with religious response to such medical issues. I would, therefore, like information addressing the Jewish belief on the issue of organ transplants. Can you also address the issues of willing organs to science as well as carrying donor cards? Your help on this matter is much appreciated and I look forward to hearing from you.

Answer: I propose to divide the discussion of organ transplants into three parts: the requirements of *halakhah* (Jewish law), a general discussion of the principles involved, and examples of rabbinic opinion, giving a small sample of the in-depth consideration the subject requires.

1. *Halakhah*

Jewish law requires that the organ donated must be potentially life saving and should not be donated for the purpose of general experimentation or research. Even when this requirement is met, the collection of the organ must be carefully monitored. It must be done with due regard for dignity and respect for the body that housed a soul. The collection must be strictly limited to what is needed. What is not needed must be replaced for burial, even if it must be removed temporarily to harvest the organ desired. The body must be draped for the sake of modesty and respect as if in an operation, and there should be no levity during the procedure.

It is therefore important for someone who wishes to donate an organ or organs to arrange that the next of kin be made fully aware of their wishes, and that the next of kin consult with proper rabbinic authority when the times comes.

The ordinary donor card is, therefore, not acceptable. Instead, a carefully worded written document should be drawn up and witnessed. It should be in the care of the next of kin or whoever will be in charge of arrangements after death.

To maintain this standard Judaism prefers that a "health-care proxy" be appointed. He or she will make decisions in extremis or after death, but only with rabbinic consultation. Health-care-proxy appointment forms are available through American rabbinic and lay organizations.[7]

2. Principles

Certain general principles of Jewish medical ethics apply.[8]

The first principle is the supreme sanctity of human life. As the story of creation unfolds, we find that the Almighty creates a world even for only one person. Imagine how worthy man is in the eyes of God. To Judaism, human life is not, as other faiths regard it, of immense importance, but rather of infinite importance. The difference determines the Jewish view in many matters connected with death and dying, donation of organs, and transplant surgery.

The *Compendium on [Jewish] Medical Ethics* summarizes the major points. In transplant surgery two values are paramount, the needs of the recipient and the rights of the donor. The needs of the recipient are matters of life and death. Almost all laws of Judaism give way before this. Under those circumstances it is not only permitted, but commendable to make use of an organ of a corpse, and it is considered a merit, not a desecration.

But one value that does not and never can give way is the

---

7. The Rabbinical Council of America has such a form. The Union of Orthodox Jewish Congregations of America encourages its use. The Agudath Israel, a lay organization with Rabbinic backing, has a similar, though slightly longer form. Either would be acceptable.
8. Chapters dealing with this subject are to be found in Rosner, *Modern Medicine and Jewish Ethics* (1986), Rosner and Tendler *Practical Medical Halakhah* (1990), Jakobovits, *Jewish Medical Ethics* (revised edition New York 1975), and Tendler in his transcribed lectures given in Australia, *The Tendler Lectures* (Sydney, 1987), and in *The Yearbook of Medical Ethics, Jews' College*, (London, 1993), the latter two edited by N. Shulman.

right of the donor. One may not shorten his life by even one instant. The time of death is, therefore, immensely important. One may not even prepare a critically ill person for the operation to remove an organ before he dies lest it hasten his death by an instant. If human life is infinitely important, then time doesn't count before infinity. A moment of life is as important as a lifetime. So it is necessary to determine the exact time of death, and Judaism is very much concerned with that. Much has been written on the subject.[9] These issues will be discussed in greater detail below.[10]

Based on the principle that each human life is of infinite value, is the Jewish belief in the equality of man. The Talmud declares that another message of man's having been created alone is that "One person shall not say, 'My father is better than yours.' Are we not all children of one human being?"[11] Indeed, if each of us is of infinite value, then one person may not be in another's service. God says, "You are my servants, not servants unto servants."[12]

So we may not sacrifice one life for the sake of another, even when the saved person is granted many more years of constructive living. If we violate this law, it is considered murder. The supreme duty to save human life is to result in a net gain, not a trade-off. Do not substitute one life for another. If we are of infinite worth, then we cannot put price tags on anyone. We cannot even assess the value of two people as being higher than that of one person. Infinity is infinity.

Supposing someone made a will saying his vital organ

9. *Compendium on [Jewish] Medical Ethics* (Federation of Jewish Philanthropies, New York 1984), Sixth edition, ed. Rosner and Feldman, p. 67.
10. See Infra, pp. 135–145, dealing with the ethics of cardiac surgery, especially the summary of opinions on the subject of the moment of death in the response to Dr. Glenville by N. E. Shulman.
11. Talmud Sanhedrin 37a.
12. Talmud Kiddushin, 22b; cf. Lev. 25:39–43.

should be offered even before he dies? Obviously this must be disregarded. We cannot contribute a vital organ to another, even if the decision was made without any coercion whatsoever. It is forbidden by Jewish law. You cannot forfeit your life to save somebody else's, because you are not in charge of your life to forfeit it. So the donation of a vital organ while the donor is alive cannot be accepted.

However, in considering the risk versus benefit ratio, we find a different story. Judaism allows a person to take a small, reasonable risk to achieve great benefit. But he or she must be totally free to make that decision without coercion. Two examples are given in the Jerusalem Talmud that can be put in modern terms as follows. Someone is drowning in your swimming pool. Extending a long pole to him will save his life. There is no risk to you. Then not to put out the pole is a passive act of murder. Another case, however, is quite different. There is a storm off the beach. A fisherman's boat founders. You are a good swimmer. Should you jump into the ocean and swim out to him? Will you reach him? Will he pull you down? There is some doubt and therefore some risk. In this case you cannot be blamed if you decide, instead of swimming out to him, to run for help.[13]

The third principle, that the human being is created in the image of God, requires us to afford respect in life and in death. Thus it is forbidden to derive benefit from the bodies of the dead or to desecrate them. Burial must take place without delay. Every part of the body must be buried. For man's creation in the image of God requires that every possible measure of dignity be extended to the human body in death as in life. That is why the body must be regarded as inviolate.

For that reason, Jewish law does not sanction the perfor-

---

13. The development of this discussion follows Moshe D. Tendler in a lecture given in Australia at St. Vincent's Hospital, "When Not to Treat," *The Tendler Lectures, First Sydney Conference on Jewish Bioethics*, August 11–19, 1987 (ed. N. E. Shulman), pp. 31ff.

mance of autopsies except to save life. A post-mortem may therefore be performed to gain specific information of benefit in the treatment of other patients already afflicted by a life-threatening disease. A case in point would be a person who has died after receiving an experimental drug, or drug combinations, that had been administered to a group of patients.

Even so, autopsy cannot be performed if the deceased had objected, or if the immediate relatives refuse permission. The dominant consideration in permitting an autopsy is the immediacy of the constructive application of the findings. With modern communications, such findings can have life-saving effect almost everywhere in the world.

But even when permitted, the autopsy must be done with great respect to the deceased. It is therefore to be done as a surgical procedure with the same dignity, respect and consideration that would be accorded a living patient undergoing an operation. It should be in dignified surroundings. The patient should be draped as normally in surgery with only the area of the incision exposed. The procedure should be done with proper decorum. The autopsy should be limited to the derivation of the information needed for saving life. Permission to use the body to save life does not grant permission to do additional procedures for any other purpose. That would be a desecration of the dead.

Organs should, therefore, not be removed from the body, but examined in place, except when the information cannot be obtained in any other way. Even then, all organs must be returned to the body for burial, except for small sections necessary for microscopic examination and for pathology "blocks" as required by law. All organs and body fluids must be returned for burial.[14]

Thus, we see how Judaism stresses that body and soul belong to God. The answer to the question, "Whose body is it

14. See Rosner, *Modern Medicine and Jewish Ethics* (New York 1986), pp. 277ff.

anyway?" is "God's." This answer affects more than autopsy. It affects abortion, the right to die, to will parts of my body away, to meddle with it, change it, transmute its sex, decorate it with tattoos, and so forth. The Jewish answer is that the body, like the soul, belongs to the Almighty. It is not ours to change, harm, or damage, or treat it however we wish to do. The Yom Kippur prayer declares: *Haneshama lach, vehaguf paalach,* "Soul and body are Thine."[15]

The body is given to us in trust. We are to tend it, but we cannot harm it, since it belongs to Almighty God. What happens when we can no longer care for it? It reverts to another steward, the next of kin. Supposing there is no next of kin, or they are not available? Then the nearest person becomes the representative of society and is obligated to care for the deceased.

Once we are aware of these principles we begin to perceive the consistency of Jewish answers to other medical issues of today.

I may not commit suicide. I may not hurt myself. I must not even cut myself, except for therapeutic purposes. No permanent engraving may be made in skin or flesh, such as a tattoo. May I will part of my body to science? Not for experimentation, but yes, indeed, if it will save a life, provided I do not endanger myself thereby.

After my death, I may give vital organs as well. During my lifetime, may I give a non-vital part of my body away? Yes, to save a life, but only because saving life takes precedence over the prohibition against meddling with my body, and provided it is a small risk for a large gain.

Corneal Transplants

In obtaining the cornea from a deceased individual for transplantation to a blind recipient, the biblical prohibitions of

---

15. See Yom Kippur prayers, *viduy,* confession of sin, at the end of the *Amida.*

deriving benefit from the dead, desecrating the dead, and delaying the burial of the dead are all set aside because of the consideration of saving a life, *pikuach nefesh*. For blindness is considered by most rabbinical authorities to be a life-threatening illness because of all the dangers to which such a condition exposes the victim. Most rabbinic authorities extend this to include even the loss of sight of only one eye.[16]

All transplanted organs, including the grafted cornea, become an integral part of the recipient.

It is permissible to donate one's eyes to an eye bank even if a specific recipient has not yet been identified. There is always a shortage of donated eyes, and therefore a reasonable certainty that they will be promptly used in life-saving (i.e., sight-restoring) operations.

Kidney Transplants

Is the donor allowed to subject himself to the danger, however small, of the surgical removal of one of his kidneys in order to save another's life? One is obligated to avoid all danger to one's physical well-being. Nor is one permitted to wound oneself intentionally. Nor may we set aside one person's life for the sake of another.[17] So may one endanger

---

16. The late Isaac Yehuda Unterman, of blessed memory, then Chief Rabbi of Israel, in a classic responsum written in *Responsa Shevet Miyehudah* (Jerusalem 1955), pp. 313–322, wrote that in bone and nose transplant there is no *pikuach nefesh* (life threatening illness), so other prohibitions such as desecration of the Sabbath or deriving benefit from the dead such as through transplant, cannot be set aside. But there *is* such a consideration in connection with sight loss and eye transplant, for a blind man is in physical danger of harming himself at any time. Eye transplants would therefore take precedence over almost all prohibitions, so that Sabbath restrictions would be set aside and transplant of corneas from cadavers would be permitted.
17. Mishnah Ohalot, 7:6; Maimonides, Mishneh Torah, "Hilchot Rotzeach Ushmirat Hanefesh," 1:9; Karo, Shulchan Aruch "Yoreh Deah" 425:2.

one's own life by donating a kidney in order to save another's life? The Jerusalem Talmud concludes that one is obligated to place oneself even into a possibly dangerous situation to save another's life. It seems logical that the reason is that the kidney recipient's death without intervention is a certainty, whereas the donor's is only a possibility.[18]

On the basis of this passage, Chief Rabbi Emeritus Lord Jakobovits has ruled that a donor may endanger his own life or health to supply a "spare" organ to the recipient whose life would thereby be saved only if the probability of saving the recipient's life is substantially greater than the risk to the donor's life or health.[19]

Rabbi Eliezer Yehuda Waldenberg discusses at length the question of whether a healthy person must, or merely has an option, to donate one of his organs for transplantation to a desperately ill individual in order to save the latter from certain death. He concludes affirmatively, if doctors certify that there is no danger to that individual, and if the donor is not coerced into acceding to the procedure.[20]

Most Rabbinical authorities assert that it is permissible but not obligatory, because the probability of saving the recipient's life is substantially greater than the risk to the donor's life or health. This principle is applicable to all organ transplantation where live donors are used as a source of the organ. A small risk may be undertaken by the donor if the chances of success for the recipient are substantial.

---

18. This principle is found in commentaries on Maimonides Mishneh Torah "Hilchot Rotzeach . . ." 1:14, and Rabbi Joshua Falk Cohen, SEMA, Shulhan Aruch "Hoshen Mishpat," 426:1, and later codes Aruch Hashulchan, 426:4, in nearly identical language.
19. See Jakobovits, Jewish Medical Ethics (New York 1975), p. 290f. Cf. Rosner, loc. cit., who cites a personal communication from Lord Jakobovits for this opinion.
20. Eliezer Waldenberg, Responsa Tzitz Eliezer, Vol. 9, No. 45, (Jerusalem 1967), pp. 179–185.

Thus, although wastes can be eliminated by hemodialysis, when both kidneys are diseased life is considered threatened, and transplant is permitted. The use of cadaver kidneys is permitted because in life threatening illness all prohibitions to use an organ of a dead donor are set aside.

Question: I am writing on the issue of kidney donation, because as the nephrologist in Bradford I have been asked by transplant physicians in Leeds to address the problem of cadaver kidney donations from Bradford patients. You will be aware of the national shortage of kidneys for transplantation.

Answer: Kidney donations from cadavers are permitted. Kidney transplant is a life saving operation, and a Jewish person may, even should, donate life-saving organs to save the life of others. While a Jew is prohibited from desecrating a dead body and may not derive benefit from it, this does not apply to life saving situations as in the case of kidney disease. In that case, use of organs from the deceased to save a life is considered a great merit for the soul of the departed.

According to some authorities of Jewish law, use of cadaver kidneys has become more desirable than live donor kidneys. Moshe D. Tendler states that nowadays the chances of rejection of a cadaver kidney have been so greatly diminished by new drugs that success figures are almost as impressive as with a live donor kidney. On the other hand, it has been found that life with one kidney carries additional risks of diabetes, high blood pressure illnesses, and the like. He is, therefore, of the opinion that a cadaver kidney is preferred to a live donor organ.[21]

---

21. He gave this opinion in a *Jerusalem Post* interview, June 10, 1987, and later confirmed it in personal conversation with me.

This ruling would apply only if cadaver kidneys were readily available. England has a shortage of such kidneys. In such a situation there is no choice but to sanction the use of a voluntarily offered kidney from a live donor. In a group discussion I once wondered out loud why in England there is such a shortage of cadavers for organ donation. Someone suggested that it was because England does not have liberal gun laws and is therefore a far less violent society than the United States. Be that as it may, until there are enough cadavers to satisfy the demand for kidney donations, voluntary donation from live donors will still be permitted by Jewish law.

Tendler adds that when organs are donated by transplantation, a Jew has no priority over a non-Jew. "Priorities in allocating organs must be established solely on the basis of medical suitability and then either by random selection or on a first-come first-served basis. Any critera based on social worth threaten the ethical foundations of a democratic society." [22]

What about the burial of an organ removed from the body of a human being? A small amount (the size of an olive) of flesh from a deceased requires burial. Tissue or blood removed from a living person does not. A limb removed from a live person requires burial, even though it is small, such as a little finger, providing it is comprised of flesh, tendons and bone. This might exclude organs removed at transplant, such as a heart, gall bladder, stomach, or lung. Nevertheless, there are rabbinic opinions that require burial of whole organs removed in surgery for other reasons, such as: 1. The prohibition against deriving benefit from parts of a human. 2. The possibility that ritual defilement would be caused by contact with such an organ. 3. A human body is compared to the parchment of a scroll of Torah that requires burial should it no longer be usable. In this respect there is no difference be-

---

22. In an interview with Judy Siegel, staff writer for the *Jerusalem Post*, June 10, 1987, Israel edition (Vol. LV No. 16543), and later confirmed personally to me.

tween an entire Torah scroll and one letter. So, too, part of
the body should be respectfully buried. Sensitivity to the feelings of a religious person would therefore indicate the need
for burial of such boneless organs as well.[23]

23. Y. M. Tukechinsky, *Gesher HaHayim* (Jerusalem 1960), Part I,
Ch. 17:2, pp. 143–146, summarizes, indicating that a limb, be
it ever so small, such as a child's finger, must be buried. A piece
of tissue the size of an olive, when it is from a cadaver, must,
according to some opinions, be buried. Blood which issued after
death or shortly before death in the amount of a reviis (app. 3
and 1/3 oz.), must be buried. When a limb was removed during a person's life, it must be buried. It is washed before burial.
If a person objects to burial of the limb during his lifetime,
some opinions hold that it can be preserved until the death of
the person and buried with him. Teeth which fell or were removed from a cadaver after death require burial. If they were
removed during life they do not require burial.

Cardiac Surgery: Ethical Dilemmas

Question: Transplant surgery becomes more complicated when faced with issues raised by cardiac surgery. For many medical dilemmas in different areas of medicine converge. For instance, what would Judaism say about selection of patients for transplants? Who does the selecting? What about issues concerning the right to know? How much must any doctor tell his or her patient, especially when the patient must theoretically share in serious decision making, such as when a person decides to undergo heart surgery and possibly transplant? What about the allocation of scarce resources, such as intensive care beds? Every surgical discipline requires that kind of support, and when the resources are limited, who wins the space and on what basis? And who decides who will be released from intensive care and on what basis is such a decision to be made?

Answer: All of these issues are, as you say, intertwined. One of the best analyses of The Doctor's Dilemma is made by Dr. Simon L. Cohen in his book, *Whose Life is It Anyhow?* It is a book written "in an attempt to inform the public of the ethical dilemmas encountered in intensive care treatment."[24] Dr. Cohen has spent more than twenty years as physician to the Intensive Care Unit at University College Hospital in central London. It is all the more pertinent to our discussion since the author is an observant Jew who tries, as much as he is able, to apply Jewish Medical Ethics to the constant daily dilemmas he faces. In it he discusses most of your questions, including such dilemmas as who qualifies for intensive care, when to stop, withholding and withdrawing intensive care, decisions about resuscitation including whether it is right to keep a patient, already brain-stem dead, on a ventilator only in order to harvest his or her life saving organs, autonomy, euthanasia, and, almost climactically, transplant ethics. I refer you to this wonderful book for answers to those of your questions which can be answered, and add the following quotation from the book, since it is obviously one of Dr. Cohen's guiding principles which he enunciates in the words of Rabbi J. David Bleich. He writes:

> Rabbi Bleich, Professor of Jewish Law and Philosophy at Yeshiva University, New York City, has summarized the Orthodox Jewish position by pointing out that the proprietor of all human life is God Himself and that man is but a trustee of his life. The concept of sanctity of life supercedes considerations of personal freedom. Were autonomy the paramount value, society would not shrink from sanctioning suicide, mercy killing, even consent to homicide. Bleich adds that, according to Jewish ethics, casting off the yoke of the law is not an act of freedom but its antithesis.[25]

---

24. Simon Cohen, *Whose Life is It Anyhow?* (Robson Books, London 1993).
25. Ibid., p. 145. His citation is from J. D. Bleich, "The Moral Obligation of the Physician," *Doctors' Decisions* (Oxford University Press, 1989), ed. G. R. Dunstan and E. A. Shinebourne, pp. 13–27.

Your perceptive questions will find resonance in that excellent book. Some of them will be echoed in the following section in which I include the transcript of a public discussion between a cardiac surgeon and myself.

Question: Cardiac surgery presents new ethical problems and raises serious halakhic issues, such as when is a patient really dead, and how do we allocate scarce medical resources. Rabbis are still discussing certain important issues presented by such transplants, particularly the problem raised by the fact that the heart is useless as a donated organ if it is allowed to stop beating for more than a very brief period before harvesting.

Answer: Following is an edited transcript of a program that took place at the Centre for Medical Ethics, Jews' College, London, consisting of a lecture by Mr. Brian Glenville,[26] cardiac surgeon, a rabbinic response by myself, and excerpts from the ensuing discussion.[27]

Mr. Brian Glenville on the Ethics of Cardiac Surgery

Cardiac surgery is a very young practice. The first valve replacement was done only three decades ago, the first heart transplant, only twenty-five years ago, and coronary bypasses became successful and popular only in the 70s. Large strides have been taken in a short time.

When looking at the methods and ethical principles that have driven the surgeons, one wonders how progress was made at all, or that those who made it were not locked up

---

26. In Great Britain surgeons are called "Mister" rather than Doctor.
27. The lecture and discussion are reprinted with permission from the 1993 *Yearbook of The Centre for Medical Ethics, Jews' College*, London, Patron, Lord Immanuel Jakobovits, ed. N. E. Shulman.

for manslaughter before they had produced their results. Most current procedures are well established today. We know that there is a favorable risk and benefit profile for many of the more common operations. That was not true for the early attempts at these procedures.

How do we go about developing new operations, particularly in congenital surgery? There are few animal models. The fact remains that whatever one thinks of it, many of the new operations for congenital heart disease are devised in the theater on the human patient for the first time. Currently that is the only way to develop operations which at the end of the day are crude plumbing. Nonetheless, the plumbing has to be worked out and the connections have to be seen to work in practice.

Even in adult cardiac surgery, there in no such thing as the perfect valve replacement. If an aortic or mitral valve replacement is needed, we are faced with making the appropriate choice to replace the malfunctioning original. Almost every year new valves appear on the market. There is a choice from over one hundred and fifty. These valves need extensive testing to get an FDA license for implantation. The real testing, however, is done on the human model, and that has some important ethical implications as to whether one would choose to use the latest technology or stick with what is tried and tested, in which case you may actually be doing your patient a disfavor.

The same applies to conduits. We hear about bypass grafts. Something like ninety-seven percent of all patients undergoing coronary artery bypass grafting come through the operation very well, provided they survive the surgery. We are interested in patients not only getting out of the hospital but also deriving some benefit and seeing whether they have an increased length of life as well as a decrease in their angina. For many years we used saphenous veins, and that served very well. We know that the veins themselves have a ready attrition rate. They block up, and patients return with recurrent angina and a second operation is more risky. Other conduits have been developed, such as the left and right internal mammary artery, the gastro-peploic artery, and a variety of other conduits to try to overcome the problem of veins. Do these have other complications of which we do not know? Is the risk greater?

There is, of course, the continual problem that nearly all of the decisions we have to take in our daily practice are genuine life and death decisions for our patient, and consequently very difficult for the practicing surgeon to make. As the only Jewish cardiac surgeon in London, I do not have any peers with like attitudes with whom to discuss many of these problems.

Progress must be made. How else will surgery achieve new techniques, new valves, new conduits, and new approaches? Is it ethical for a surgeon to practice in this way? Is it ethical for a Jewish surgeon actually to participate in an experimental procedure before the outcome is definitely known? Now, twenty-five years after its inception, I can give you quite respectable survival results for cardiac transplantation. It will generally be agreed that it is an ethical operation to perform. But, somebody had to start in 1967 when the outcome was unknown. What would we think is ethical, if this lecture were taking place in 1966 rather than now? Those are issues I am forced to deal with not only in a theoretical, but in a very practical way.

I have daily ethical dilemmas. I am interested in building a strong department and am busy politically, lobbying for cardiac surgery in order to obtain the largest share of "the cake." Every pound I manage to squeeze out is taken away from somebody else.

Even within the department we have a finite budget. We measure the costs to the National Health Service which is on the order of three to four thousand pounds for a vein graft and nearer eight thousand pounds for a valve replacement. Coronary Artery Bypass Graft (CABG) is cost effective. Almost regardless of the age of the patient, that operation will be paid back to the state somehow, within two or three years. A young working man of 45 will repay the operation within a year and a lady of 75 will still repay the operation if she survives three years, which she is likely to do. She will be taking less medication, requiring less in the way of social services, and so forth.

Valve replacements, however, are not cost effective. They are less successful. They are more expensive. They very rarely pay themselves back. Now, considering our fixed budget, how do I set the proportion of valve patients? Shall I slant my budget to favor valve patients, thus doing an injustice or at least a great disservice to a large number of CABG patients, who would not only have benefitted, but actually would have paid their operations back in a short time? Or shall I favor the CABG procedure because of costs? It is easy to say "treat everybody on their merits." But life is not like that. We have fixed budgets and are presented with large numbers of patients. We are forced to set priorities.

This brings us to the waiting list and its structure. When patients are put on a waiting list we are taking a best guess as to how long that patient can survive without surgery. We are forced into the position of actually doing our best to assess a patient clinically to see how long it would be ethical and safe to allow him to wait. A common problem is deciding between a patient who continues to smoke and one who has done his best to control risk factors. Am I to give them equal priorities, or can I treat them on positive merits? Can I warn a patient, saying, "If you don't stop smoking, I'll put you at the end of the waiting list"?

What about informed consent? Cardiac surgery is so highly specialized that not even other doctors, let alone patients, are in a position to decide what type of valve, or repair, or replacement, or refinement of procedure should be used or done. As for me, although I ask my patients to sign an informed consent form, I suggest to you that "informed" means "exactly what I want them to know." In truth, I hope that they rely on the fact that their doctor is genuinely trying to do what is in their best interest. But it is not, in the true sense, "informed consent."

Planning for intensive care is also a problem. We have a fixed number of beds, and if I do not plan my week in a fairly

crude and harsh manner, I will not be able to practice. If I
operate on an 83 year-old who needs a double valve replacement, she will occupy an intensive care bed for five days. If I
select that patient for a Monday, her bed will not be available to me until Saturday. If I perform that operation on a
Friday, there is a good chance that I might be able to get her
to a High Dependency Unit on the following Monday. If so, I
will be able to carry on with the list. If I operate on a Monday,
I am stopping four CABG patients, who would have zipped
through on Tuesday, Wednesday, Thursday, and Friday.

The result is that when I am called on a Sunday night with
a very urgent referral, I do everything that I can to postpone
the operation until the end of the week. I find this difficult
to defend ethically. If I do not practice this way, however, I
will get very few operations done. Globally, the situation would
be quite appalling.

Long before Christian Barnard, the concept of heart transplantation was discussed. The mechanics of heart transplants
involve a number of ethical issues. The first thing to do is find
the donor. This is a problem in the UK, since the number of
donors offered for transplantation is about two thousand a
year. Even if more patients are encouraged not to wear crash
helmets when riding motorcycles and not use seat belts when
driving, that number may not rise sufficiently. So we really are
dealing with a fixed population.

So what happens? A donor is found and we assess a variety of parameters to decide whether that particular offer of
organ donation is going to be suitable for us. We look at our
list for an appropriate recipient who would benefit from this
particular heart. We then travel to the donor's hospital and
one of the many things we do, apart from assessing the
donor's physiological state, is to see whether proper protocol
has been followed to determine that the donor is dead. Two
independent doctors who are not part of the transplant team
performing the operation and equally not concerned with the
people offering the heart, usually neurologists or anesthetists,
have independently, and on two successive occasions separated

by a respectable time interval, gone through the criteria that we now accept for brain stem death. At that point, the patient is on a respirator and being supported. If the heart actually stops beating, it is not usable. We can take the heart only when it is still beating. We take it and preserve it in much the same way as we preserve a heart undergoing surgery. It is very easy to stop a heart, but it is a nice trick to make it work again at the other end. At that stage we prepare the recipient but do not open the chest until the procedure is well progressed, and we do not remove the diseased heart until the new heart is physically in the same operating theater.

What are the issues? At one time they raised the problem of double murder. Was the donor really dead? Did the recipient really have a reasonable chance of survival? Did the recipient really have a chance to give informed consent? Today the question is whether it is "single murder." Is the donor dead if his heart still beats? But the recipient certainly has a good chance. The recipient success rate is ninety percent of patients alive at one year, in excess of seventy-five percent alive at five years. The figures are quite respectable. There are a number of conditions, including cancer of many organs, where a seventy-five percent five-year survival is not attained. Most of our patients enjoy a high quality of life and live relatively normal lives, although they do take a great deal of medication.

It is one thing for me to tell you about my experience today. It is entirely different for those who pioneered it. The ethical problems that they experienced were really quite extreme. But Maimonides' principles for following new techniques are equally valid today. He said "Anything proven effective in practice, even though one could not understand how it worked, or something that followed from a rational deduction based on a generally accepted physical theory, is ethical and right to continue." I find that a useful way to think.[28]

We do have many problems in choosing recipients. Most

---

28. Maimonides, *Commentary to the Mishnah*, Talmud, Yoma 83a, Chapter 8, *Mi sheachazo bulmus.* . . .

patients fall into two major categories. In one category are those with end-stage ischemic disease, who have had major heart attacks and are not suitable for revascularization by conventional technique, since the heart muscle is too badly damaged to survive surgery. In the other category are the cardiomyopathies where the heart muscle, for reasons that we do not understand, has given up the ghost, and they have gone into severe intractable pump failure. Most of the patients selected would normally be dead within one year. Our continued controls are the patients who do not get transplanted. There are exceptions to that rule, and some people do recover. We have to have age criteria because of the limited donor pool as well as criteria of size and weight.

Who actually is empowered to do the choosing? Should it be the head of the transplant service alone? With whom should he consult, or should he play The Great Deity himself? These are important issues to be addressed. And once we decide who should do the choosing, the final question is, whom to choose. These are all ethical problems that I have both the good and bad fortune to have in my daily practice.

Response

Cardiac as well as general surgery take risks and benefits into account. There is the major concern of the hazard of the surgery itself. In transplant surgery there is also an equally great concern that the rights and integrity of the donor be safeguarded.

It is a truism in Judaism that the imminence of death in no way compromises the inviolable rights and privileges of the donor. One who is extremely ill has the full protection of the law. Shortening his life by one second is an act of murder. It is therefore categorically prohibited to prepare a critically sick donor for transplant surgery if this preparation in any way hastens his death. One is prohibited from touching or moving a *goses*, one who is about to die, lest one inadvertently hasten his or her death.[29]

Cessation of spontaneous respiration and absence of a heartbeat for a given time period represents the classical Jewish legal interpretation of death. But, of course, in heart transplant cases heartbeat must be continued artificially if the donor heart is to be usable.

Dr. Glenville raised the issue of experimental surgery. A scandal erupted in August 1988 involving Dr. Michael Bewick, a surgeon, who leaked an experimental effort to the press involving the use of pig organs for human transplant. In the ensuing public outcry and panic, Dr. Bewick was forced to resign. There is, in Jewish tradition, an opinion that the reason it is forbidden to eat pig is that of all the animals its internal organs most resemble those of the human. Be that as it may, in Dr. Bewick's case, if the homework had been done and pig organs had been found suitable, there should have been no halakhic objection to using them even for non-life-threatening purposes. You are, after all, not eating them. But we are worried about the risk–benefit ratio of such procedures. Did the researchers do all their homework before contemplating human application? Is it *refuah bedukah*, a tried and tested remedy?

Obviously, if risk versus benefit is to be taken into account, then the greater the certainty of the fatal alternative, the greater is the risk allowed and the more latitude permitted for experimental surgery. It must, however, be *refuah bedukah umenusah*, sound medical protocol and not quackery.[30]

It is therefore important to distinguish between medical experimentation and medical cure. If the transplant offers a chance, even if a slim one, that is scientifically acceptable so that this is not a matter of a "wild shot," then it is permitted

29. Bab. Talmud, Tractate Semachot, 1:2, Shabbath 151b; Rambam, Mishneh Torah, Hilchot Avel, 4:5; Joseph Karo, Shulhan Aruch, Yoreh Deah 339.

30. Jacob Emden, *Mor U-Ketziah*, "Orach Chaim" 328, indicates that a patient is required to accept therapy, but only if it is of proven efficacy, a *"refuah bedukah."*

if the alternative would be near-certain death. But if there are two ways to do it and medical history shows one way is better, a doctor could not be permitted to use the less viable method.

Israel's late Chief Rabbi, Isser Yehuda Unterman, claimed that heart transplant is an exception to the normal consideration of risk versus benefit. He required heart surgery to have better than a fifty percent chance of success in order to be permitted. He reasoned that, when a person's heart is removed in the process of the operation, that person loses his *hezkat hayim*, "presumption of being alive." This was said at a time when such surgery was indeed experimental. Nothing demonstrates the flexibility of the *halakhah* system more than such a change in medical statistics, which renders that consideration moot, since the success rate is now far better than fifty percent.[31]

---

31. Five year survival figures are now 75% or better. Rabbi Unterman's view that heart transplants may not be halakhically sanctioned until such time as the chances for survival from the surgery are greater than those for failure seems to be contrary to the pronouncements of earlier rabbis (cf. Chaim Ozer Grodzinski, Achiezer, Yoreh Deah, Ch. 16) who permit greater risks in the face of greater danger. Rabbi Unterman explains that the recipient of a new heart is in a different situation from all other desperately ill, but not necessarily dying people. After his diseased heart is removed, and before the new heart is implanted, the recipient has lost his *hezkat hayim*, "presumption of still being alive." Once he loses his *hezkat hayim*, the heart transplant recipient is no longer permitted to risk his life if the chances of success are not greater than the chances of failure. A person dying of cancer, on the other hand, never loses his *hezkat hayim* and therefore may subject himself to any risk, however great, if there is a small chance for cure. The definition of *hezkat hayim* is illustrated in the Talmud (Gittin 28a) where it states that: "If a messenger brings a divorce document from a distant place, and the husband was old or sick at the time the messenger left, he should still deliver it to the wife on the presumption that the husband is still alive." Thus, unless we have positive information to the contrary, a person retains his *hezkat hayim* until pronounced dead.

Triage

A far more serious problem facing us in radical surgery is the issue of selection. (See response to Mr. Glenville on page 143.) The most serious problem of the '90s is scarce resources in money, space, beds, machinery, surgeons, organs, and so on. And of course, in the real world, one makes priorities. May we? Dare we?

Daniel Callahan is director of the Hastings Center and a leading biochemist. Dr. Tendler said that Callahan's book, *Setting Limits*, can be reviewed in one sentence. "If you are past 75, you have had it."[32] Callahan's point of view makes us wonder about setting priorities. Consider the verse about healing in Deuteronomy that Maimonides likes best. "You are obligated to heal the sick patient, because if he lost his donkey you must return it to him. *Hashev teshivem*, 'return his lost property' (Deut. 22:1). How much more must you return his lost health." Nowhere does it say you do not have to return an old donkey, or heal an old man, or cure an old woman. Age-related considerations were not factored into God's re-

---

32. "The Tendler Symposium," *Yearbook of the Centre of Medical Ethics, Jews' College*, 1993, p. 105.

quirement to heal. Any attempt to use such considerations in order to differentiate between our obligations to one segment of society and another runs counter to the direct instructions of the Torah.

Dayan Berger, past member of London's Beth Din, indicates that priorities exist. He outlined, for example, that when a woman and a man both desperately need food, a woman takes precedence over a man because it would be less dignified and more shameful for a woman to go begging than a man.[33] A woman is ransomed before a man if both are captives,[34] but a man takes precedence over a woman if both are drowning.[35] The Talmud enumerates additional priorities.[36]

Not everyone agrees. In life and death situations, *mai hazit dedamach didach sumak tefey*, "why do you consider your blood redder than your neighbor's"?[37] In fact, there is a halakhic view that we dare not set priorities. For that was the bedrock of Nazi medicine, which set priorities about age, mental state, social worth, quality of life, state of health, and, ultimately, race.

At a Mount Sinai Hospital Medical Ethics Symposium, the following was reported:

> The questions were brought to a head during the Holocaust. There were a variety of tragic questions like those concerning redemption of individuals and selection of individuals. Rabbi Shimon Efrati, Rabbi Tzevi Hirsch Meizel, Rabbi Efrayim Oshri all wrote Holocaust responsa based on death camp experiences. For example, in Auschwitz on the eve of Rosh Hashanah the Nazis rounded up 1400 boys chosen to

---

33. *Shulhan Aruch, Yoreh Deah* 251:8, and "Sifse Cohen" commentary ibid. See also Mishnah Horayoth, 3:7.
34. Ibid.
35. Ibid., see "Ture Zahav Commentary" on 252:8.
36. Mishnah Horayot 3:7 and Bab. Talmud Horayot, 13a, 13b, and 14a. *Cf.* Rabinovitch, N.L., "What is the Halacha for Organ Transplants," Tradition 9(4):20–27, Spring 1968.
37. Bab. Talmud, Pesachim, 25b.

be killed. Parents tried to redeem them. They asked, "Is it possible to redeem or ransom them from the authorities, knowing that someone else would be killed in their place?" The Rabbis referred to the rule, "Who said that your blood was redder than your neighbor's, or that your child's blood is redder than that of his child?"

If Meizels and others, ruling out of the depths of the night, contravened the Mishna in *Horayot*, what shall we say or do? Can we establish one person's worth over another's?[38]

Many authorities say we cannot choose. We must accept either such principles as first come first served, or random selection, or a lottery, or some other arbitrary measure. Rabbi Moshe Feinstein was asked about eight meningitis patients at the Hadassah Medical Center. Penicillin had just arrived, but there was only one dose, enough for eleven injections. Without even thirty seconds' hesitation, he answered, "The first bed the doctor comes to."[39]

Even so, Dayan Berger claims a distinction between Holocaust selection—which the Nazis tried to force us to perform as part of their program to deliberately dehumanize us, and that therefore we had to resist at all costs—and a system of priorities that in any case must be set.

There is no argument that choices must be made. There is a great deal of opposition to succumbing to social pressure that perceives some as worth more than others, whether because of contribution to society, age, quality of life, number of dependents, sex, marriage, intelligence, race, or any other criterion.

Yet in the real world there are finite resources, and what can we do? There is some help in a Talmudic discussion of community versus individual concern. Rabbi Moshe D.

---

38. Marc Gellman, *Mt. Sinai Journal of Medicine, 50th Anniversary* issue, Jan. 1984, Vol. 51, No. 1, p. 115.
39. Moshe Feinstein, *Responsa Iggrot Mashe*, No. 251.

Tendler developed the idea in a Mount Sinai Medical Center Symposium and later for the *Jews' College Yearbook of Jewish Medical Ethics*:[40]

> The Talmud rules that paying an exorbitant amount of money to redeem a captive is forbidden. The Talmud explains this fatalistic attitude in two opinions, one based on the reasoning "lest society be impoverished," the other on "lest ransom encourage the kidnappers to increase their attacks." The first line of reasoning is that society cannot afford ransom; if we were to ransom these people, we would not have money for other social needs, and, therefore, we can only extend our sympathy. It is a classic triage. The second line of thought is that if the ante for kidnapping is high, people who never thought of kidnapping would start: if you can get enough money robbing banks, who has to work?
>
> However, the Talmud says that a husband can redeem his wife at any price and a father can redeem his son at any price. The underlying meaning is that no one can establish an ethical principle that compels society to pay any price to redeem a captive, and society can survive such an ethical decision to forgo ransoming someone. But a husband has a duty to his wife to redeem her at all costs. A father may redeem his son at an exorbitant fee. Ethically, he can't be stopped from ransoming, because basically he is doing what is correct. He says that money does not count when it comes to saving a life. Here you see a clear distinction between a societal ethical decision and a private ethical decision. Society needs money for other expenditures.
>
> This is so despite the fact that the Talmud underscores that there is no greater *mitzvah* [good deed] than ransoming

40. Moshe D. Tendler, "Rabbinic Comment: Triage of Resources," *The Mount Sinai Journal of Medicine*, Vol. 51 Number 1 (January-February 1984), pp. 106ff, and *The Yearbook of the Centre for Medical Ethics, Jews College*, London (1993), p. 157.

someone who has been captured. Surely it is a *mitzvah* to feed the hungry and the thirsty and clothe the naked? Someone who is a captive has all these needs combined. Redeeming him is a multiple *mitzvah*. Yet society is forbidden to spend an extra dollar. Society cannot afford it.

The concept of relative need in society is developed in a second example in the Talmud. A town on a hill was successful in digging a well and a town lower down was not. Of course there is moral obligation on the town above to provide water for both towns. You cannot let the other town die. If the higher town had only enough for itself, then the town below should move. If the town above had enough for both only if they refrained from laundering their clothes, then the Talmud rules that the town above should wash its clothes and not provide water to the lower town. Why? Because in the long run, it is impossible to survive without washing your clothes. The immediate danger is to the lower town. The long-range danger affects both towns equally. Typhus would certainly decimate the higher town in time if no one washed their clothes.[41]

Society differs from the individual in the time scale that it uses for decisions. An individual responds to the problem at hand. Society has a long-range view. Society must deal with its future survival. Of course, each individual should worry about the future of society, but the individual's decision-making process concentrates on the here and now. The long-range view must be taken by society.

Triage decisions are made between two communities: I have water, you don't have water. They are made between two departments: who gets the allocation of funds? But triage

---

41. Talmud *Nedarim* 80b; 81a. Rabbi Yosi establishes the principle that it is impossible to survive without washing clothes. His view is not to be viewed as a singular opinion, but as an elucidation of the discussion of the Talmud. It can therefore be accepted as a halakhic norm.

decisions between our generation and those yet unborn must also be made. A classic case of intergenerational triage is evident in plutonium technology. Even with all our technology, we do not yet know what to do with radioactive waste. We could say, let us put it into cement canisters, dump it in the ocean. We have enough technology now to hide waste certainly for five hundred years. But what happens after that? What about the yet unborn generations? After five hundred years, how many people will get leukemia and how many will have malformed children? Whose concern is this? Do triage concerns extend to other generations? Of course they do. The individual must place the immediate problem of saving life first. Society can be excused if it considers the future first.

Finally, of special concern in this whole analysis is the domino theory, also known as the slippery slope of medical ethics. Unfortunately, societal decisions can sometimes lead to amorality. Dr. Leo Alexander,[42] writing after his return from the Nuremberg trials, commented on how it was that German medicine became the basis of immorality. How could it have degraded the human organism as never before? It was a time of triage. There was not money for everybody. That is how it started; Germany was in financial stress. The first medical decision was not to treat the incurables. That decision, Alexander says, ended up as: do not treat anybody who disagrees with me. The next decision was: kill everybody who disagrees with me.[43]

Given a set of priorities, preferably set by the hospital and not by the individual physician, and given the assumption that highest or very high on that priority list is the patient who already had the procedure and has now relapsed, may the

---

42. Alexander I. "Medical Science Under Dictatorship," *New England Journal of Medicine* (1979, 241:39).
43. Moshe D. Tendler, "Medical Ethics Conference," *Yearbook of the Centre for Medical Ethics, Jews' College*, London, p. 157f.

individual doctor remove a patient from such a high priority if the damage done is his own fault? May a doctor warn a patient with the words, "If you persist in smoking and it causes you a setback, I call that suicide and I don't want to know you. You'll wait till the end of the line." After all, such patients who do not heed their warnings are harming themselves. Do they forfeit their place? Admittedly, one must try to prevent suicides. But shall they retain a high priority on the list?

The issue could be compared to a responsum in the *Kometz Minchah* commentary to the *Minchat Hinuch*[44] as to whether someone is required to intervene to halt an attempted suicide. The *Minchat Hinuch* cites the three requisites for healing: *rapo yerape*, that a doctor may practice his art; *vehashevoto lo*, that we are required to restore a person's lost health just as we are required to restore his lost object; and *lo taamod al dam reecha*, "Do not stand by doing nothing when your neighbor's blood is flowing." Not only does the finger point at us requiring that we heal, but we are required to undergo expense—one sage says even a modicum of risk— to save him.[45]

Whereupon *Kometz Mincha*'s commentary adds the following: "It appears prima facie that, if someone is attempting suicide, and another can save him but fails to do so, then he surely would not be violating the requirement of returning his lost health, just as, should someone throw his possessions away, the finder is surely not required to return them to him."[46] He further suggests the possibility that even the prohibition against standing by while your neighbor's blood flows should not apply. Rabbi Meir of Rothenberg, known as *Mahara'm*, disagrees.[47]

---

44. Mitzvah No. 237.
45. Supra, p. 14.
46. Kometz Mincha, Responsa, "Shulchan Aruch, Choshen Mishpat," No. 10.
47. Responsa of Meir of Rothenberg, Responsum, No. 39.

I discussed the matter with Dayan Berger, who feels that the doctor is justified when threatening to withhold treatment, and that such a warning when issued can be carried out, because a warning without teeth is no warning.[48] Needless to say, there are those who agree with Rabbi Meir of Rothenberg, who requires that we intervene to help in such a situation as well.

---

48. He bases his view on the Kometz Mincha cited above, and on the Talmud, "Shabbat 4a," referring to Tosafot, loc. cit., which distinguishes between a person who transgresses purposely and one who does so accidentally, after a warning.

Informed Consent

One of the important issues raised by Mr. Glenville (see page 143) is that of informed consent. The issue is not limited to cardiac surgery. It can easily be divided into two areas of inter-action: the truth telling of a diagnosis; and the sharing of the responsibility for the treatment to follow.

In *halakhah* we say all requirements of Jewish law give way to the primary requirement to save life, *pikuach nefesh*. Tell-ing a lie is morally wrong. But it is not murder, adultery, or idolatry, the three sins you must avoid on pain of death. To save a life you tell a lie.

In America, the right of privacy and the patient's right to know are related. In effect, the patient is entitled to know any information that anyone else knows about him. This makes it very difficult to prevent the patient's discovering information about the state of his or her health that could be discourag-ing. In fact, in recent years, physicians have been disclosing to patients possible consequences even more dire than they themselves assume to be the case, for they are often in the defensive position of doing whatever is necessary to avoid being vulnerable to law suits. On the other hand, the religiously observant physician, as well as the family, are obligated to avoid causing the patient to become depressed, and this is very often hard to reconcile with the absolute truth.

For the *Code of Jewish Law*, "Hilchot Bikur Cholim" No. 383, introduces two concepts: "It is forbidden to tell [a critically ill patient] that which will "break his heart or upset his mind"; in other words, things that will cause depression or cause him to give up his will to live.

The Jewish approach to patient who is seriously sick is to inform him that many have survived this illness, so he should not lose hope, but the illness is grave and therefore whatever is necessary to "set his house in order" physically and spiritually, should be done. Under such circumstances, the tact of the physician is severely tested. How does the physician inform the patient of the seriousness of his illness without causing him to lose hope of survival?

The issue becomes less difficult when it comes to discussion with a patient modality of treatment. The *halakhah* would require sufficient disclosure to enable the patient to make a completely informed decision. This does not mean the patient must know as much as the doctor. Rather, he must know enough to make an informed decision to trust or not to trust the doctor with the surgery. Too much technical information might be counterproductive, serving only to confuse or depress the patient. The patient does not want technical details either. He does want to hear the doctor's advice and must know enough to decide whether to trust the doctor enough to undergo the proposed procedure willingly. If his illness is serious, he needs to know it, but, where possible, must be aware that his case is not hopeless.

The differences between the Jewish and general approach derive from a fundamental difference between the *halakhic* approach to medicine and a secular approach. We speak of medicine as citizen's rights. You are entitled to medical care, for you are a taxpayer and citizen. Hence, it is a battle between rights: the right of a physician not to treat; the right of a patient to seek treatment; the right of any individual to obtain what he wants in life.

Halakhah operates with obligations rather than rights. There are duties, *mitzvot*, religious obligations. There is the obligation to treat, even at some risk or expense; and the obligation to take care of your body which does not belong to you, but to God who entrusted it into your care.

The "patient's right to know" is often equated with "patient autonomy." Why do I have the right to know everything possible about myself? Because I have a right over my own body. Autonomy requires that we be able to dispose of our own bodies, treat or mistreat them as we see fit, even commit suicide. "Not so," says Judaism. "*Haneshama lach vehaguf paalach*," "Soul and body are Thine."

The resultant attitude of Judaism is that every part of the healing team must strive to heal as an obligation. The doctor has an obligation beyond that of a mere contract with patient. The patient has an obligation to tend the body given him in trust by the Almighty. Society has an obligation to see that healing proceed in the best way for the most people. And if in the process, the patient's right to know is partially diminished for the sake of effecting a cure, and even if only for the sake of easing their suffering, then the obligation to partially withhold the depressing and hope destroying information takes precedence.

The Moment of Death

The most important issue of all is the question of the moment of death. (See response to Mr. Glenville on page 143.) The criteria for the determination of total destruction of the brain were set forth by Harvard University's Commission appointed to do so by the US government. The criteria are as follows:

The Harvard Criteria

Brain death, according to the President's Commission's report, known as "The Harvard Criteria," is defined as total cessation of all brain functions, including the cessation of independent respiratory control. A neurological definition of death must include abolition of function at cerebral, brain-stem, and perhaps even spinal-cord levels. The Harvard criteria of death include "irreversible coma" as part of the neurological definition of death. These criteria are unreceptivity and unresponsiveness to externally applied stimuli, even intensely noxious stimuli; no spontaneous muscular movements or spontaneous respiration (spontaneous respiration is tested by brief removal from a mechanical respirator with monitoring of blood and even carbon dioxide tension); no reflexes; an isoelectric EEG (tested at high gain); the tests are to be repeated at least twenty-four hours later with no change. Hypothermia and central nervous system depressants must be excluded as causative factors.

These criteria are accepted by most universities in America as criteria of death. A patient with brain-stem death who meets all the so-called Harvard Criteria for irreversible coma would, at autopsy, show histological evidence of what pathologists term "respirator brain."

Following is a summary of major Jewish scholars' opinions.

Rabbis Feinstein and Tendler

As Mr. Glenville pointed out, at the very beginning of the period of heart transplants, more than twenty-five years ago, Rabbi Feinstein and Israel's Chief Rabbi, Isser Yehuda Unterman, forbade the practice, calling it "double murder." The donor and the recipient were both considered victims of murder. As we know, Rabbi Unterman elucidated that the patient loses *hezkat hayim*, presumption of life, as soon as his heart is removed.

Rabbi Tendler wrote a responsum that he summarized in the Jews' College Medical Ethics Center Conference in 1993. His words had earlier been quoted in the *Jewish Observer* of October 1991, as follows:

> Brain-stem death does not mean that the brain died and the body lives. It is not analogous to cardiac failure or liver failure, which is the failure of an organ. The *Mishnah* (*Ohalos* 1:7) instructs us that anatomical decapitation (actual removal of the head) results in halakhic death of the entire body even though the heart still beats and the limbs twitch. The Talmud (*Chulin* 21a), in its statement *Zikna Shaani*, concludes that anatomical decapitation (actual removal of the head) is not an absolute requirement. Even if no external wounding occurs, if the connection . . . between the brain and body is interrupted, the entire body is dead, i.e., there is organismal death. Therefore a *kohen* may not enter the room. It is for-

bidden to transgress the Sabbath for such a "cadaver," and there is a duty to bury the body. The clinical picture is described by Rashi in *Yoma* 85a, referring to a man buried under rubble on *Shabbos*: if he appears clinically dead, if he does not move his limbs, how much do you dig to determine the truth? The Talmud concludes "until you expose his nose" so as to determine whether he makes any respiratory efforts because "the source of life is in the breath."

Brain-stem death that is determined after careful neurological examination affirms that the following criteria of death are all present: completely unreactive pupils, no spontaneous or elicited eye movements, no motor response to stimulation, no grimacing, blink response, gag response, and no respiratory movement, cough, sigh, or hiccup, confirmed by an apnea test in which the patient is hyperoxygenated prior to disconnecting the ventilator.[49]

Rabbi Moshe Feinstein wrote four responsa concerning determination of the time of death. In three of these he clearly refers to the type of patient now known in medical literature as Karen Quinlan or Nancy Cruzan cases. He clearly defines his patient as *yachol linshom*, "capable of breathing independently." This is not a brain-stem-dead patient but one referred to as cerebral dead, PVS, or locked-in syndrome. Such a patient is entitled to full medical care. In his fourth responsum on brain-stem death, Rabbi Feinstein identifies the condition as follows: "the doctors put him on a ventilator so that he breathes even though he is dead. Such breathing does not qualify to consider him alive."[50]

Dr. Mordecai Halperin, Director of the Ethics Department of Shaare Zedek Hospital in Jerusalem, has defended Dr. Tendler's position in his writings. So has Dr. Rosner.

---

49. Bleck, T. P. and Smith, M. C. "Diagnosing Death and Persistent Vegetative States," *Journal of Critical Illness*, 1989 4(11); 60–65.

50. Iggrot Moshe, "Yoreh Deah" Vol. III, Res. No. 132.

Rabbis A. Soloveitchik and J. David Bleich

Rabbi Aaron Soloveitchik holds that death is an ongoing process and is not complete until all organs no longer function, including the heart, and so he precludes heart transplant altogether. He reasons from Maimonides, who declares: "If the brain . . . spills like water . . . the animal is a *treifah* (unable to survive; lit. "torn").[51] Since by definition a *treifah* is alive, reasons Rabbi Soloveitchik, it follows that an animal or human being is regarded as still alive even though the brain has liquified.

Rabbi J. David Bleich agrees with Rabbi Soloveitchik, and argues that mere cessation of blood flow to the brain is not the halakhic equivalent of decapitation. He further argues that if respiratory activity is regarded as the sole determining criterion of the presence of life, it would follow that a polio victim who is entirely dependent upon an iron lung machine or a similar device in order to live would be regarded as dead despite the fact that such an individual is fully conscious and is indeed capable of engaging in intellectual activities requiring a high degree of cognition. He also argues that in the light of the halakhic prohibition against moving even the limb of a *goses*, a dying patient, lest the patient's death be hastened thereby, it would be difficult to perform testing procedures upon a moribund patient without violating applicable halakhic strictures.

Rabbi Joseph B. Soloveichik

Rabbi Tendler writes about Rabbi Joseph B. Soloveichik's view as follows:

> Although a student of Hagaon Horav Yoseph Dov Soloveichik, of blessed memory, for almost half a century, I cannot recall a clear *psak* [legal decision] from him on this issue. I can

---

51. *Code of Jewish Law*, Hilchot Shechitah, 6:4.

recall numerous conversations in which his only expressed reservation was to the accuracy and reproducibility of the testing protocol.

I would also add that the *Rav* established as Rabbinical Council of America policy to support all halakhic decisions of the Chief Rabbinate of Israel that are of international, not local import.

Rabbis Herschel Schachter and Eliezer Waldenberg

Rabbi Schachter, also of Yeshiva University, indicates that life is defined by heartbeat and not by respiration. Lack of breathing merely indicates the lack of heartbeat. Rabbi Eliezer Waldenberg of Israel agrees with this point of view.[52] He wonders why Rabbi Moshe Feinstein, in his responsa, ignores the question of heartbeat. He opposes the view of Rabbi Tendler, saying that "if we accept the opinion that the death of any one of the vital organs defines the person as dead, it might result in some rather startling conclusions. If a person's liver is removed, or, according to Rav Moshe Feinstein's understanding even if it is gangrenous, although that person can still walk, talk, and think, he would be considered halakhically dead!" He therefore accepts the idea that a person is not considered dead until all the vital organs are dead.

Rabbi Jakobovits and the London Beth Din

Rabbi Yitzchok Yaakov Weiss of Manchester strongly condemned cardiac transplants.[53] Lord Jakobovits, then Chief Rabbi, had written to Rabbi Weiss that a transplant operation

---

52. Eliezer Waldenberg, *Responsa Tzitz Eliezer*, Vol. IX, No. 46; Vol. X, No. 25:4.
53. *Hamaor*, Brooklyn, Part 5, No. 178, Elul, 5728, [Aug.-Sept.] 1968, pp. 3–9.

may require artificial extension of the donor's heartbeat and respiration by the use of a respirator until the recipient can be prepared to receive the new heart. As a result, the following halakhic question arises: is it lawful to ventilate the brain-dead donor artificially solely to preserve his heart long enough to effect the transplant, and, having done so, is it lawful to then shut off the respirator, thus, in effect, seeming to manipulate the life and death of the donor at will? This question that the Chief Rabbi believes is relevant to the whole problem was answered negatively by Rabbi Weiss, while Rabbi Auerbach of the Kol Torah Yeshiva in Jerusalem offered an affirmative reply.

Rabbi Aryeh Leib Grosnass of the London Beth Din wrote that a person would still be considered alive by Jewish law if his breathing were maintained by artificial means.

Lord Jakobovits' son, Dr. Yoel Jakobovits of Baltimore, had published a letter to Rabbi Tendler, saying "Without doubt your interpretation of Rav Moshe's written word can be firmly supported. Your personal knowledge of Rav Moshe's thought processes make you the likely expert. However, I believe Rav Moshe's written statements are not unequivocal and are therefore open to interpretation. I remain puzzled as to why, on such an important issue, this should be so." And in a letter to Rabbi Tendler, Lord Jakobovits declares, "I read it all carefully but I am still unconvinced." Lord Jakobovits himself wrote to Rabbi Tendler to say, "On brain death as well as on organ transplants and living wills, opinions are clearly still deeply divided, and it would be idle for me to pretend otherwise. . . . Respecting your opinion does not and cannot prevent me from recognizing that there are other [opinions] too."

Rabbi Elyashiv and Others

Rabbi Yoseph Elyashiv did not accept brain stem death. Originally, he issued the following statement together with Rabbi Shlomo Zalman Auerbach: "It is our view that it is absolutely forbidden to remove any of [the patient's] organs [on the basis of brain-stem death alone], and to do so would involve taking a life."

Rabbi Tendler indicated that an experiment had been conducted in Israel, concerning a gestating sheep, that Rabbi Elyashiv was watching with the possibility of changing his mind. That experiment was a success. "Nevertheless," Rabbi Tendler reported, "Rabbi Elyashiv had said the matter needs further study."

The Chief Rabbinate and Transplants

Responding to a 1986 query from the Health Ministry on the subject of heart transplants, the Council of the Chief Rabbinate in Israel addressed the issue of the moment of death as follows:

> Based on the Talmudic principles enunciated in Yoma 85 and [ruled accordingly in Responsa] Hatam Sofer in "Yoreh Deah" 3:338, *halakhah* holds that death occurs with cessation of respiration. This can be established by the confirmation of the destruction of the entire brain, including the brain stem that is the pivotal activator of independent respiration in humans.
>
> It is accepted in medical circles that this requires five conditions: definite knowledge of the etiology of the brain damage, complete cessation of natural respiration, detailed clinical verification of brain-stem destruction, objective and established scientific tests of brain stem destruction such as BAER, and clear evidence that this condition has continued for at least twelve hours in spite of continued intensive care.
>
> In the light of the forgoing, the Chief Rabbinate of Israel is prepared to authorize heart transplants (from motor vehicle victims) at the Hadassah Hospital under the following conditions: all the aforementioned conditions are met, a representative of the Chief Rabbinate is a full member of the committee that establishes donor death. The Ministry of Health will choose him from a list submitted annually by the Chief Rabbinate, consent by the donor or next of kin is obtained

in writing, a committee of review is set up to oversee that the conditions are met, the Ministry of Health is to supervise and insure that these conditions are universally maintained throughout the land.

Essential criteria for the establishment of brain death include very strict medical tests confirming a state of deep coma and absence of independent respiration, clear evidence of structural damage to brain tissue not subject to therapy, non-treatable structural damage to brain tissue, . . . absence of any type of autonomous convulsions, absence of brain stem reflexes, oculo-cephalic (doll's eyes) pupillary light reflexes, corneal, vestibular ocular (caloric) testing with ocular instillation of ice water in the absence of outer ear occlusion, non-response of the facial muscles to deep somatic pain, cough or gag reflexes.[54]

The controversy is far from over, but, of course, if we are to allow heart transplants we must accept the view of the Chief Rabbinate of Israel and Rabbi Tendler, citing his revered father-in-law, Rabbi Feinstein.

Rabbi Chaim Zimmerman

Finally, a note from Rabbi Chaim Zimmerman

Definitions of death keep changing with the steady advance of scientific knowledge throughout the generations. On the other hand, axioms of *halakhah* and its definitions never change. Only circumstances of their application undergo change. From a practical point of view, we are seeking not the definition of death, but rather the definition of LIFE. For as long as the person is alive there is the *mitzvah* of *pikuach*

---

54. As reported in Barkai, Spring 5747. Dr. Yoel Jakobovits translated and commented in Tradition, 24(4), Summer 1989. The translation is largely my own, but relying on that of Dr. Yoel Jakobovits for the technical sections.

nefesh [saving a life] and there is also the prohibition of *retzicha* [murder]. If a person can be brought back to life, he was definitely never dead. He is a *chai lekhol davar*, "living in every respect." Whoever kills him is culpable. We come now to a definition of life. "As long as there is any quantitative functioning of life observable in a human being *baolam hazeh*, in the realm of our mundane life, he is alive."[55]

Discussion

A number of important questions were raised in the discussion.

Question: The point of view that focuses on heartbeat as the determinant of life or death raises many logical problems. What does one do when the patient goes on to bypass? If the man is a *kohen*, does his wife's status become in doubt as soon as he goes onto artificial circulation? Is she a temporary widow? What about the inheritance of his property? There are many logical inconsistencies.

Answer (Rabbi Shulman): Dr. Rosner lists those questions that you raised and adds several more, including the possibility that after the removal of the old heart and prior to the implantation of the new, the surgeon might be guilty of murder! There are many such questions, and the answer to all of them is that the criterion is whether we are seeking to save life. No one says that the heart alone is the source of life. The Talmud says it is respiration. The question remains, is it respiration with or without a heart?

---

55. Chaim Zimmerman, "Life as a Relative Concept in Halacha," Intercom, Vol. XI, No. 1, Jan. 1970.

Comment (Dr. Glenville): Wherever we are, we are faced with the overriding concern about the lack of resources. I have practiced in the States, where they also have to do the best with their resource limitations. We have diversities all over. In China, where one is led to believe the society is incredibly egalitarian, matters are even worse than in the States. If a farmer cannot afford to pay for his heart operation, he is not hospitalized.

Question: Allocation of scarce resources is the key issue. If the community can prioritize, can we have explicit rationing determined by the community? With regard to the 75-year-old female with the CABG, I suppose we as general practitioners are your feeder mechanism. I have never yet had such a patient referred even for angiography, let alone bypass grafting. The rationing has gone on before they ever got to your level.

Another point that you may have answered: is it permissible to be able to pay for life-saving treatment when it is not obtainable through the Health Service? Should the ability to pay be a criterion? Angiography is available in forty eight hours, bypass in a week, in the private sector. On the NHS, angiography has a waiting list of four to six months, and the waiting list for bypass grafting is usually a year or more. Of course, while they are waiting, they may die.

Answer (Mr. Glenville): I cannot answer the ethical side. I am sure you are right in what you say about all of the 75-year-olds out there who might be referred but are not because you do not think it is appropriate. Perhaps I should not be telling you this, but there are plenty of people who do think they are appropriate, and I did three such patients in the last week. The average age of our patients is remarkably high. It is a question of rationing. It happens to be one operation that you can actually justify. I have tried to separate the ethical from the cost effective, although you are linking them yet again in a global sense with regard to budget. These operations are cost effective at almost any age. Therefore, however you share the cake on an individual or on a community level, this is one type of operation that one can ethically justify for almost any age group dependent on their medical needs and not their social or economic circumstances. If you were asking this question concerning valve replacement operations, I would be on much stickier ground. We tend not to accept very old patients for valve replacements unless there is a good expectation of improving them.

Answer (Rabbi Shulman): As far as payment is concerned, if a person can pay for an operation and does not pay for someone else to get off of the list, of course he can go to private medicine. That is the rationale of the private medicine service.

Comment: If they are ordinary outpatients, they are never referred onward if they are over 70. There is a cutoff.

Question: Would Judaism agree with my own personal political view that if someone can afford to have treatment privately, then they should have it privately, thus releasing a bed for someone who cannot afford it? Have you made a distinction in the status of patients between the taking of the donor organ and the actual implanting of this separated organ into a recipient?

Answer (Rabbi Shulman): Rabbi Feinstein says that the object of removal of the heart must be to place it with a given recipient.

Comment: If the heart has already been removed, and the Jewish patient is not going to benefit, then someone else will benefit.

Answer (Rabbi Shulman): Judaism makes no distinction between Jewish and non-Jewish donors and recipients.

Question: If we accept the definition of brain-stem death, and therefore it is not murder to remove a beating heart from a brain-stem-dead patient, is there any halakhic ruling on who can be a donor? I was given to understand that one should not touch a body after death has been proclaimed, that it is a mutilation to remove the heart. Is there any *halakhah* on that?

Answer (Rabbi Shulman): It is a *mitzvah*, fulfilment of a commandment, to donate organs. God commands we do whatever we can to save life. Everybody agrees that this applies even to eyes and other such organs. With the heart, there is a special issue of the moment of death, but every other organ except the liver, can be harvested after death. However, you should not carry the kind of donor card that gives a blanket permission to have all organs donated.

5

Organ Donation and Health Care Proxy

Question: As a counselor working in a children's hospital, I am only too much aware of the need for transplanted organs and tissue to save life. My husband and I feel we should donate our organs or other parts of our bodies after death if they could save life or restore a quality of life such as is possible with a corneal donation. What is the halakhic attitude to such organ donation? Is this permissible?

Answer: I commend you on your intent to save life through transplantation, once life is over. No Divine and human service, no mitzvah, is greater than saving life. The commandment to save life supercedes the prohibition against marring the body of a deceased or deriving benefit from it.

Of course, a vital organ may not be donated before life is over. Afterwards, it must be done in conformity with Jewish law, and therefore the usual donor cards are not permitted. Instead, a proxy could be appointed who would carry out your wishes in consultation with rabbinic authorities, insuring that the organs are indeed used exclusively to save life, and not for training, anatomy classes, or any other purpose.

The Rabbinical Council of America has a detailed form for appointing a "Health Care Proxy." So does the Agudath Israel organization of America. Some rabbis in England consider these forms to be cumbersome and unnecessary. They feel that if a proper proxy is appointed who knows you well and is informed of your wishes, and if proper Rabbinic and medical consultation is carried out, the decisions based on specific conditions of illness can be made at that time. If you truly trust the proxy and have conveyed what you have done to your next of kin, then the medical details need not be fully anticipated. The appointment note should state clearly that every decision of life or death should be made only with rabbinic consultation.

Jewish law considers corneal transplant to be life saving.

May you live a long and healthy life; so long, that eventually your organs will grow to be far "over-age" to be of any use. . . .

Living Will

Question: I would like to donate my organs to save life after my death. What is Judaism's view about the Living Will? Is this the right way to do this?

Answer: Judaism is against the Living Will as it now appears in the documents proposed to patients. There are many reasons for this.

The Living Will is based on a patient's absolute right to dispose of his body and body parts. It presumes a person's right to terminate his own life. Many who accept these premises are nevertheless opposed to the Living Will for such reasons as the following:

1. Since it is difficult to determine whether death is imminent, the Living Will provisions may be activated prematurely.
2. Evaluation of medical or surgical procedures as merely death-postponing rather than life-prolonging is often arguable. Methods considered heroic and of only tempo-

rary death-postponing value have, with the advance of
medical science, proved to be life-sustaining.

3. During the five-year period when the Living Will is usually in effect, a patient may change his mind and yet
   not formally rescind the declaration, thus leaving the
   Will to be activated without proper informed consent.
   (Medical evaluation has clearly demonstrated that many
   patients do change their minds when faced with the actual decision of life or death.)

4. The existence of this Will could deprive the patient of
   full concern by the medical team, who might not otherwise pursue treatment with the greater level of care
   demanded by the patient's condition.

5. Pain appears to be the major symptom justifying the ac-
   tivation of the Living Will. But medical science has begun to explore in depth the field of pain relief, as well
   as the special role of the hospice for the terminally ill.
   The Will would deflect attention and effort from forms
   of pain relief and encourage withholding of life-prolonging treatment.

6. There are no strict criteria to differentiate between a
   critically ill and a terminally ill patient. How terminal
   is terminal? Is it to be measured in days, weeks, or
   months?

7. The doctor's moral conscience or religious convictions
   may be compromised when his actions are restricted by
   the terms of the Living Will.[1]

In addition to all the above arguments, Judaism objects to the
very premise of the Living Will, believing that our body is not
our own but belongs to the Almighty. It is given to us in trust.
We may neither harm it nor destroy it. We have no right to

---

1. Summarized in the *Compendium on Medical Ethics*, Sixth Edition, 1984 (Federation of Jewish Philanthropies of New York),
   130 E. 59th Street, N.Y.C., 10022. Pages 115–117.

terminate our lives, nor may we instruct others to do so. Judaism, therefore, does not support the use of "Living Wills" by patients, nor reliance on such documents by physicians.

On the other hand, patients who want to donate organs after death, or who want their wishes expressed in case of terminal illness in a situation where they may not be able to convey them, can appoint a Halakhic Health Care Proxy. This differs from the "Living Will" in that the proxy is required to consult with rabbinic as well as medical authorities, and the decision will be based on conditions existent at the time the inquiry is made, while taking the wishes of the patient into account. The Rabbinical Council of America as well as the Agudas Yisroel have suggested appropriate forms for this. Some British rabbis are of the opinion that detailed anticipation of possible terminal conditions is not necessary in advance. A general halakhic proxy appointment would be sufficient. Judaism therefore opposes a Living Will document, but does not oppose a document appointing a trusted person as a health-care proxy, provided that it requires all decisions in critical situations to be made according to halakhic law and stipulates that there be consultation with halakhic authorities such as a rabbi or rabbinic court judge at the time of decisions in matters such as withholding treatment, disconnecting life support machinery, autopsy, or organ donation. The rabbi or member of the Beth Din would, after full consultation with the medical team and the family, be able to provide the Jewish view on the condition at that time, taking into account medical as well as halakhic requirements.

Euthanasia

Question: One of the most important current issues is euthanasia and the problems arising from our ability to artificially prolong life. Can you respond to this? Can you give your opinion of the paper written by Dan Brock, Professor of Philosophy and Biomedical Ethics at Brown University who writes in favor of euthanasia?

Question: Could you furnish me with a statement on whether, according to Judaism, tubal feeding may be removed from a comatose patient?

Question: Sometimes prolonging life is actually prolonging the dying process. What does Judaism say about this?

Question: Can you address the issue of "physician-assisted suicide?"

Answer: Dr. Dan Brock, Professor of Philosophy and Biomedical Ethics and Director of the Center for Biomedical Ethics, Brown University, Providence, Rhode Island, wrote a paper in favor of euthanasia since, as he indicated, "no issue in biomedical ethics has been more prominent than the debate about forgoing life-sustaining treatment. Controversy continues regarding some aspects of that debate, such as forgoing life-sustaining nutrition and hydration. . . ."[2]

While the conclusion of his study is in favor of voluntary, active euthanasia, he is careful to claim that:

1. There is no difference between passive and active euthanasia. . . . The belief that doctors do not in fact kill requires the corollary belief that forgoing life-sustaining treatment, whether by not starting or by stopping treatment, is allowing to die, not killing. Common though this view is, . . . it is confused and mistaken.[3] One kills when one performs an action that causes the death of a person (we are in a boat, you cannot swim, I push you overboard, and you drown), and one allows to die when one has the ability and opportunity to prevent the death of another, knows this, and omits doing so with the result that the person dies (we are in a boat, you cannot swim, you fall overboard, I don't throw you an available life ring, and you drown). [They are one and the same.]

2. Patients who cannot give consent themselves because they are in coma are also free of pain and may not be afforded euthanasia. "The determination that the patient is incompetent means that choice is not possible."[4]

3. Modern science has learned how to control . . . pain, so that pain, if properly treated, can be overcome.

2. Dan W. Brock, "Voluntary Active Euthanasia", *Hastings Centre Report*, March-April 1992, Vol. XXII No. 2, p. 10.
3. Ibid., p. 12.
4. Ibid., p. 13.

How does Judaism regard these issues?

I was asked to address this subject at a Conference on Death and Dying sponsored by the College of Physicians of Edinburgh. The following reply is excerpted from the full paper that was published in their "Proceedings."[5]

Three important guiding principles of Jewish medical ethics that apply to the subject of death and dying, are: the human being is possessed of a unique dignity since he is created in "the spirit of Godliness," or, as is often translated, "in the image of God"; one's body is not one's own, but lent by God in stewardship; human life is of infinite importance. In the light of these principles, let us consider how Judaism regards the process of dying.

Jewish tradition views death as inevitable and just. A Jewish legend, cited in the Talmud, tells of a sage who managed to steal the sword of the Angel of Death. He though he would do humanity a favor by eliminating death. The Almighty commanded him to return the sword, saying, "My creatures need it." Death has its place in God's plan for this world.[6]

Jewish law requires the physician to do everything in his power to prolong life but prohibits the use of measures that prolong the act of dying. This is a fine distinction, and, as Lord Jakobovits pointed out, often very difficult to maintain. Consequently, the question arises, till when shall we treat?

The Divine license by which the physician pursues his calling is limited to healing and the prolongation of life. Faced with the inability to do that, the physician must declare with honesty and humility, "I have done my best." He then steps down from the stance of physician and becomes a caring human being, friend, counselor, and skilled easer of pain. In

---

5. N. E. Shulman, "Prolonging Life, Prolonging Dying," *Proceedings of the Royal College of Physicians of Edinburgh* (June, 1990, Vol. 20, Number 4) pp. 427–433.
6. Talmud, Ketuvoth 77b.

such a situation, "curing becomes caring."[7] But though hope may be gone, a physician may not shorten life even by a moment. A patient with but a moment to live, has all the rights of a healthy individual.

Thus the major problem of the physician under his Divine license to heal is what happens when he comes to the end of his ability to cure. The following are broad guidelines:

1. When death is otherwise a certainty, high-risk procedures may be accepted by the patient, but not at any risk. The decision must be based on sound medicine. The attitude "what have I to lose?" is not defensible on moral grounds. A very high risk is permitted for a commensurately high potential benefit.[8]

2. A patient who suffers from an inexorable terminal condition with no possibility of cure is nevertheless entitled to all basic life-support maintenance and therapy such as food, liquid, and intravenous infusion when necessary. Antibiotics to cure infection and other such routine therapies are also required. Life-support machinery need not be instituted; some say, may not be instituted.[9]

Rabbi Dr. Moshe Dovid Tendler describes the problem as follows:

> Removing an intravenous from a patient who is not drinking will cause him to dehydrate and die in a matter of days. There is an attitude that: "After all, if he can drink, I'll let him go and get a glass of water. I'm not going to stop him." But he can't drink. "He requires that a needle be stuck into his vein,

---

7. Moshe D. Tendler, "When Not to Treat," *The Tendler Lectures, Proceedings of the First Sydney Conference on Jewish Bioethics,* (August, 1987), ed. Nisson E. Shulman. pp. 31–46.

8. Fred Rosner and Moshe D. Tendler's discussion of "Risk-Benefit Ratio," The *Mount Sinai Journal of Medicine,* Vol 51, No. 1, January–February 1984 (New York), pp. 58–64. See also *Compendium,* pp. 98–99.

9. Eliezer Waldenberg, *Responsa Tzitz Eliezer,* Vol. 13, no. 89.

and then I'll have to sterilize the water . . . that's heroic treatment!" Now it is really the way you give that patient water, and it is not at all heroic treatment. What it is, is the slippery slope.

I would like to suggest from all biblical precedents, and there are many, [removing hydration] would be looked upon as an act of murder. It is one thing not to resuscitate. That is open to discussion. I may have a different point of view than someone from another religious orientation. It is possibly acceptable not to respond even to a pneumonia by providing penicillin, where the patient is in a permanent vegetative state, and we are going no place. I repeat that I would not agree from my vantage point, but I can see the ethics and morals from the other point of view [since many patients recover from pneumonia by themselves, without treatment]. I do not know of any way to justify the removal of water and food from a patient totally in your care. It is no different from any other form of euthanasia. The fact that it is so called "passive" euthanasia is also false. I believe it is an "active" euthanasia, for "passive" and "active" are not defined by whether you push in or pull out. "Active" is whether you intervene unnecessarily or do not intervene when you must. If you have an obligation to intervene and fail to do so, that is "active" euthanasia. [10]

(As we have seen, Dr. Dan Brock, though writing in favor of euthanasia, offers a similar argument about removal of hydration and tubal feeding.) [11]

3. Relief of pain is adequate reason to assume palliative therapy even with attendant risk.

4. Pain, defined by the patient as unbearable, and which cannot be alleviated, becomes a significant reason for withholding or stopping all but the most basic maintenance

---

10. Moshe D. Tendler, "Care of the Terminally Ill," Proceedings of the Sydney Conference, pp. 39f, and pp. 47–70.
11. Supra, p. 188.

therapy, such as intravenous fluids, or oxygen. Rabbi Moshe Feinstein, who was, till his death, the Dean of the American Rabbinate and the most respected international voice in Jewish medical ethics, writes: "Certainly it is prohibited to use means to lengthen life for a short time if [the patient] will be in great pain."[12]

What about life-prolonging treatment? Is there a time when it is not indicated? Dr. Fred Rosner, Chief of the Department of Medicine of the Mount Sinai Services at Queens Hospital Center and co-editor of the *Compendium of Jewish Medical Ethics*, states: "One is not obligated or even permitted to initiate artificial life support and/or other resuscitative efforts if it is obvious that the patient is terminally and incurably and irreversibly ill with no chance of recovery."[13]

Jewish attitudes about the dying process confirm this statement. The prohibition against shortening life is expressed in the Mishnah as follows:

> One who is in a dying condition—goses—[such as can often be perceived in the last few hours of life] is regarded as a living person in all respects. One may not move him until he dies. One may not close the eyes of a dying person. He who touches a dying person or moves him is shedding blood, because Rabbi Meir used to say: "This can be compared to a flickering flame. As soon as a person touches it, it goes out. So too, whoever closes the eyes of the dying is considered to have taken his life."[14]

From this derives the principle that one may remove an impediment to death.[15] Stimuli were in use in antiquity that

---

12. Moshe Feinstein, Responsa Iggrot Moshe, "Yore Deah," Vol 2, No. 174.
13. Fred Rosner, *Modern Medicine and Jewish Ethics* (Yeshiva U. Press and Ktav Publishing, New York 1986), p. 201.
14. Mishnah, "Semachot," I, 1–4.
15. Joseph Karo, *Shulchan Aruch Yoreh Deah*, 339, No. 1.

appeared to keep the dying person alive, causing reflexes; one of these was salt placed under the tongue, another was a loud banging noise in the vicinity. A later sage declares (and his words are embodied in the Code of Jewish Law), that if a person is dying and someone near his house is chopping wood so that the soul cannot depart, then one should remove the wood chopper, in order to let the soul depart. If someone has placed salt under his tongue, remove it (even if you have to touch him to do so), because it is preventing the soul from departing the body. You may remove the impediment to death.

This can be seen more clearly in the Talmudic selection describing the dying moments of the compiler of the *Mishnah*, one of the greatest sages in all of Jewish history, the great Rabbi Judah the Prince of the second and third century, head of the Jewish community in the Holy Land at that time. "He was struggling to die," says the Talmud, "but the Rabbis who were his students were praying fervently, and that was keeping him alive." (This was either because of the sound of the prayer or because prayer is also regarded in the Talmud as a kind of therapy that is efficacious.) "His housekeeper went up to the roof and threw over a large jar, and the crash so startled the students that they stopped, giving the soul the chance to depart. The housekeeper was praised by all the Rabbis, indicating that she was right in what she did.[16] The Talmud regards the prayers of the students in that situation as an impediment to the death of their master.

However, though one may remove an impediment to death, one cannot cause death. Lord Jakobovits (1961) stated the Jewish position regarding euthanasia as follows: "[A]ny form of active euthanasia is strictly prohibited and condemned as plain murder. . . . Anyone who kills a dying person is liable to the death penalty as a common murderer. At the same time,

---

16. Talmud, Ketuvot 104a.

Jewish law sanctions the withdrawal of any factor—whether extraneous to the patient himself or not—which may artificially delay his demise in the final phase."[17] This approach has its basis in the Talmud, where we find the distinction between deliberate termination of life and artificially prolonging the process of dying. The passage describes the martyrdom of Rabbi Hananya ben Tradyon, who was the victim of the Romans during the Hadrianic persecutions of the second century.

The martyr was wrapped in the scroll of Torah from which he had been teaching and placed on a pyre of green brushwood. His chest was covered with woollen sponges drenched with water to prolong the agony of dying. His disciples urged him to open his mouth so that he might be asphyxiated and have a quicker end to his suffering. He refused to do so, saying, "Only He who has given life may take it away. No one may hasten his own death". He did, however allow the executioner to remove the wet sponges; the fire could then consume at its natural unimpeded pace. This act by the executioner of removing the hindrances to natural death was deemed meritorious.[18]

The conclusion is that a terminally ill patient may refuse certain treatments in order that his agony not be prolonged. Rabbi Hananya refused to open his mouth, because suicide and euthanasia are forbidden. To remove the wads of wool, however, is like taking away that lump of salt under a patient's tongue that they believed prolonged his life. It is called "removal of an impediment to death." Many interpret this source to teach that just as the sage allowed the wool to be removed, so is it permissible for a man whose life is of unacceptable

---

17. I. Jakobovits, "The Dying and Their Treatment in Jewish Law: Preparation for Death and Euthanasia," *Hebrew Medical Journal*, 2 (1961): pp. 251 ff. See also I. Jakobovits, *Jewish Medical Ethics*, (New York Bloch, 1959), pp. 123–125.
18. Talmud, Avoda Zara, 18a.

quality to him to request that treatment be stopped. Withdrawing all therapy would be a proper treatment for an individual who wants to die, when he is suffering intractable pain. Consequently, a terminally ill patient may request withholding of therapy in order that his agony not be prolonged.

The decision that in favor of death by withholding treatment can be made only by the patient. If an individual is not competent to make this decision because he is in deep coma, in almost all cases he will also be free of pain. If a patient is in deep coma but able to breathe without mechanical assistance, he should be afforded all the care and concern due to any sick person. The imminence of death in no way exempts the family or the medical team from fully supporting such a patient, including hydration via intravenous infusion, antibiotics when needed to treat infection, and other pharmacological agents to maintain good organ function.

Whereas a comatose patient may be a burden to his family and society, he is not so to himself, being free of physical pain or psychic trauma. Medical tests and judgments are often not sufficiently accurate to determine clearly who may benefit from continued treatment. It is better to err in favor of unnecessary continued therapy than to risk passive euthanasia. The latter could be the top of the "slippery slope" leading to neglect of patients not deemed constructive or contributing members of society.

If a comatose patient is free of pain, the family may want him to die, but the doctor may have no evidence that he wants to die. If a person is still conscious, then we judge him by what he wants. Yes, there is such a thing as "substituted judgement." But are we really so familiar with this man or woman that we can enter into their very soul and determine what their true wishes would be? We are able to do this only rarely. If there is any doubt, Judaism votes for life.

From all of the above it is clear that suicide is forbidden, and physician assisted suicide is causative murder.

Amputation and Rehabilitation

Questions: I am with the Department of Medical Engineering, King's College School of Medicine. My specialty is rehabilitation. I frequently encounter patients who had limbs amputated. I would like to know about possible emotional and religious problems I might encounter with Jewish patients, especially if they are religious.

1. Does Judaism consider amputation of a limb to be punishment for past misdeeds?
2. Does Judaism believe in resurrection of the dead? If so, would a person be resurrected with or without his amputated limb?
3. Does Judaism have any theological problem with amputation of a limb?
4. Is there any problem with an amputee participating in worship together with the congregation?
5. Might there be a problem of gender in the rehabilitation process? Is there any difference in this regard between men and women? Will Jews be reluctant to accept physiotherapy and rehabilitation treatment from a

person of the opposite gender?

6. Will Jewish families be more likely to interfere in the patient–doctor decision making process?

7. What does Judaism require to be done with an amputated limb? What should be our response if someone wants their limb preserved?

Answer: I shall endeavor to answer your questions in turn.

1. Pious Jews will try to look inward to see whether they are blameless whenever they are faced with adversity and will seek to improve their moral and spiritual condition as well as their piety if possible. This is, of course, in addition to seeking the best possible medical help. They will not necessarily blame their misfortune on previous misdeeds. They will pray for the Almighty's help in meeting and overcoming adversity.

2. We believe in the resurrection of the dead. The Almighty, who creates the miracle of birth and existence, will surely recreate whatever limbs a person lacks at the time of death.

3. We do not allow needless amputation. Amputation is permitted only for the benefit of the patient. For, after all, we are tampering with the body that the Almighty created, and He wants us to give it the respect due to that which houses the soul, the reflection of godliness. Judaism requires amputation if otherwise the patient's life may be threatened.

4. Losing a limb or part of it leads to no problems of worship in any way.[19] Once, when the Holy Temple stood on its site in Jerusalem and priests used to minister there, amputation of a limb would disqualify a priest from service. Even

---

19. See Moshe Feinstein, Responsa, Iggrot Moshe, "Orach Hayim I," nos 8 and 9, pp. 19ff, for a discussion about donning *tefilin* (phylacteries used for prayer) on a paralyzed arm and on the left hand if the right is missing.

then, neither priest nor layman would be disqualified from prayer. Since the year 70 of the present era, when the Temple was destroyed, we have no priestly service except for one Biblical sentence of blessing that the priests utter during the holiday service in synagogues outside of Israel and daily in Israel. Otherwise, the service is comprised only of prayer and Torah reading. There is, consequently, no disqualification because of the loss of a limb.

5. Rehabilitation should not present a gender problem, except in cases of pious Jews who will want to be treated by someone of their own gender. In such cases every consideration should be given to the request of the individual. If it is a matter of conscience, it must be respected. It is also psychologically helpful for the patient's positive attitude to his rehabilitation, that he or she not be burdened with feelings of guilt or embarrassment. The patient's wishes can be ascertained by the therapist with a simple query, without embarrassment to either party.

6. A family should certainly be involved in the decision to undergo serious surgery. A religious Jewish family is usually closer than a non-religious family. Families are, therefore, more likely to be involved. In many cases, a rabbi will be consulted by the patient and/or family. This is tantamount to consulting an "ethicist" and should be encouraged. The rabbi will, as a rule, encourage the family to accept the decisions of medical science, provided the surgery is not of an experimental nature, has a good chance of success, and is the best treatment for the patient's condition.[20]

7. There are, indeed, special arrangements that should be made for the burial of the limb. Every amputated limb, even a finger, must be buried in a Jewish cemetery. Usually the patient will have a plot for his or her own burial and will have

---

20. See F. Rosner, *Modern Medicine and Jewish Ethics*, (Ktav, Hoboken, New Jersey, 1986), pp. 63f. for a discussion of the family's involvement in medical decision making.

the limb buried in the very plot where he or she will eventually be buried. If that is impossible, the limb must nevertheless be buried in consecrated ground, and a Jewish burial society can help make these arrangements. This applies to organs as well. If an organ is removed from a patient during surgery, it must be buried. Pieces of tissue removed from an organ for biopsy or other such investigation need not be returned for burial.

The Jew regards the body as sacred because it is the container of the human soul, in very much the same way that the parchment of a Holy Scroll is treated with utmost respect and sanctity is ascribed to it because on it are written the holy words of God's law.[21] Thus, every part of a corpse must be buried. Even blood which has been removed from a corpse for legal reasons, such as when the body is shipped from country to country, must be placed in a container and buried with the body. Judaism is more lenient regarding a live person who suffers an amputation, requiring burial only for limbs, parts of limbs of some size, and organs.[22]

Rare instances have been known of Jews who are superstitious about burying a body part during their lifetime. In such

---

21. Babylonian Talmud, *Shabbat* 105, *Moed Katan* 25, and Nahmanides loc. cit., as cited in Gesher Hahayim; See following note.

22. Y. M. Tukechinsky, *Gesher HaHayim* (Jerusalem 1960), Part I, Ch. 17:2, pp. 143–146, summarizes, indicating that a limb, be it ever so small, such as a child's finger, must be buried. A piece of tissue the size of an olive, when it is from a cadaver, must, according to some opinions, be buried. Blood which issued after death or shortly before death in the amount of a reviis (app. 3 and 1/3 oz.), must be buried. When a limb was removed during a person's life, it must be buried. It is washed before burial. If a person objects to burial of the limb during his lifetime, some opinions hold that it can be preserved until the death of the person and buried with him. Teeth which fell or were removed from a cadaver after death require burial. If they were removed during life they do not require burial.

a case, and if they cannot be convinced to do the right thing, it is permitted to keep the limb in a preserving fluid until they themselves pass away and the limb is buried with them.[23]

---

23. Ibid.

Cryonics

Question: What does Judaism say about the attempt to freeze human corpses in preparation for a later time when science might be able to revive them? Would Judaism approve of this new science called cryonics?

Answer: Judaism has always dealt in the real world and does not consider hypothetical and "science fiction" scenarios. Until cryonics becomes a real scientific possibility, the rabbinic world will continue to give its attention to issues of immediacy in preference to hypothesis and conjecture.

Furthermore, Judaism has always considered death to be a blessing under certain conditions and in its proper time. This applies to all people. Rabbi Meir commented on the Biblical verse, "And the Lord saw everything he created, and it was very good," adding *tov meod* means - *tov mavet*,[24] "What is good about creation is death!" He did not mean, of course,

---

24. Midrash Rabbah, Genesis.

that death is good. Nor did he express a pessimistic view. After all, Judaism is very positive and optimistic in its view of life. He meant to say that one of the good things about creation was death, for it is needed.

Abraham is considered to have brought a great blessing upon the earth by stressing and teaching the values of old age. In fact, it is known that the seal of Abraham was a young man and woman on one side of a coin, and an old man and woman on the other, stressing the value of each age of life in its place.[25]

Robert Browning, in his poem, "Rabbi Ben Ezra" ("Grow old along with me, the best is yet to be, the last of life for which the first was made"), captured an essential spirit of Judaism.

I hope this gives you some sense of what Judaism's view of cryonics might be when we are ready to discuss that question and consider it.

---

25. Talmud, Baba Kama 97b.

Disaster Management

Question: (From the Board of Deputies of British Jews.) The crash of Pan America flight 190 made it abundantly clear that a master plan of disaster management must be devised. Can you provide some suggestions about the creation of such a plan?

Answer: I have had the opportunity to consult, overseas and here, with the people in charge of this area for the Israel Police Department. The following are comments I would like to suggest should be considered when making your disaster management protocol or revising it.

1. In case of disaster involving death, Jews have special needs and rules. Especially important are identification of bodies according to halakhic requirements (for agunah and burial purposes) and collection of all remains including blood and tissue for burial.

2. There are two kinds of questions: halakhic and operational.

a: Halakhic questions: Here the first line is the Beth Din, the Rabbinical Court. In all cases involving an Israeli, the matter should be transferred to the Beth Din of Jerusalem which has legal status in Israel.

b: Operational questions: Here the Israel National Police Disaster Victim Identification unit can give advice and provide operational personnel as needed. They do this on an international level without fee, except for costs of travel.

3. The local rabbi should establish contact with the families of the person or persons who have perished. He must obtain from them, in consultation and coordination with the police, a file including all the information possible to identify a person ("ante-mortem file"), including clothing sizes, dental records, medical and X-ray records, description of any scars, birth marks, fingerprints of the person if possible (on credit cards, checkbook, mahzor and other personal effects, etc). It is recommended by the Israeli Police that you use the Interpol Form for collecting the data. Using this form will standardize data since the deaths will very frequently be international, i.e., travellers who are killed away from home.

4. The British Jewish Community has responsibility for foreign Jews who are killed in disasters in this country.

5. If the Israeli DVI unit is used operationally, their invitation and utilization should be fully coordinated with the official government office responsible. The invitation should be issued by the local authority, and it is suggested that in England authority should be the Chief Rabbi's Office in consultation with the Board of Deputies. It must be coordinated with the police to facilitate their access and operational involvement. This will clarify and legitimize their status on the scene.

6. The Israel DVI unit is contacted at: Israel National Police Headquarters, Jerusalem, FAX No. 972 2 309090; Telephone No. 309493 or 309410 (Division Chief). Off hours 972 2 865797.

6

Animal Experimentation

Question (From the LYNX organization): The Chief Rabbi of Tel Aviv has, according to the newspapers, issued an order to the Jews under his jurisdiction that they are prohibited from wearing furs. One assumes he has done so for humanitarian reasons. Will the Chief Rabbi of Britain issue a similar order, likewise for humanitarian reasons? Enclosed is material detailing the cruelty in the process of fur manufacture.

Answer: Thank you for sending the newspaper reports of what the Chief Rabbi of the Sephardic community of Tel Aviv, Rabbi Chaim David HaLevi is purported to have said, and for the follow-up material which I studied carefully. I also viewed your video tape in its entirety. I agree that methods currently used to trap and kill animals for fur as you depict them, are cruel and ghastly. Surely there are better methods available for the collection of those animals required for human use.

First, let me address the question of the Sephardic Chief

Rabbi's alleged statement. Information about it is based only on newspaper report. I have taken the necessary steps to obtain the actual text of his decision. Even so, I must explain that Rabbi Halevi's ruling is limited only to his constituency, Sephardic Jews who reside in Tel Aviv. It does not apply to Sephardic Jews elsewhere, nor does it apply to any other Jewish groups. Even Rabbi Halevy's decision could not outlaw all use of animals for the sake of human-kind. He certainly would permit types of clothing, such as fur hats (most men's hats sold in shops everywhere in the world are made of animal skins), leather clothing which is universally sold and used, animals for laboratory use and for food consumption which Judaism permits, and so on.

The Chief Rabbi himself will not make any statements supporting the ban of fur manufacture or forbidding the use of animals for any of the above purposes. Animal use for the sake of human needs such as those I listed above is allowed by the Bible and Jewish Biblical tradition. But the Chief Rabbi supports all efforts to sensitize the industries concerned to the Jewish tradition and law which is very strongly opposed to causing unnecessary pain to animals. For the Chief Rabbi, and indeed all of Judaism, is unalterably opposed to wanton cruelty such as you depict in your material, or indeed any unnecessary pain caused to animals.

There are two articles in particular which express the Jewish view. I refer you to an excellent article on the subject written by Dr. Fred Rosner in his book *Modern Medicine and Jewish Ethics.*[1] Another article expressing Judaism's view is by Rabbi J. David Bleich, in his book *Judaism and Healing.*[2]

I shall summarize the most important points.

Jewish Law had many regulations designed to protect the well being of animals. Thus, the Bible commands; "You shall

---

1. Yeshiva University Press, New York, and Ktav Publishing House, (Hoboken, New Jersey, 1986).
2. Ktav Publishing House, (Hoboken, New Jersey, 1981).

not muzzle an ox while it is threshing corn" (Deut. 25:4). Placing the ox near the corn but preventing it from partaking of the food is cruel. Please note that the passage here goes so far as to forbid mental cruelty towards an animal. It does not matter that the animal does not reason. The fact that the animal has feeling is recognized by Jewish Law. Pain caused to the animal by frustrating its attempt to eat is, therefore, forbidden.

A person is obligated to provide food for his pets before he himself sits down to eat. In the same way an animal may not be overworked. Castration, spaying, sterilization of animals is forbidden under all circumstances, and a Biblical verse is cited, "And that which is mauled or crushed or torn or cut you shall not offer unto the Lord; nor shall you do this in your Land" (Lev. 22:34).

There are many other sources for the Jewish requirement to show compassion towards the animal world as well as towards fellow human beings.[3] For instance, Psalms 145:9 "His Tender Mercies are over all his Works" includes animals. Similar verses are found in 147:9, 104:14, 145:16, 36:7. In Exodus 20:10 and 23:12 we find that a person's livestock must be made to rest on the Sabbath as well as he himself.

Rosner points out that consideration for animals as a religious duty is demonstrated in numerous Biblical narratives such as when Rebecca proved that she was the proper wife for Isaac, son of Abraham the patriarch, by the fact that she brought water not only for Abraham's servant Eliezer but also for his camels (Genesis 24:14). God himself admonished Jonah saying; "And should not I have pity on Nineveh, that great city, wherein are more than six score thousand persons . . . and also so much cattle" (Jonah 4:11).

The Bible forbids the slaughtering of an animal and its young on the same day, eating of a limb cut off from a living animal, ploughing with an ox and an ass together. The Bible

---

3. Code of Jewish Law, Choshen Mishpat 426:4.

also prohibits taking the chicks from a nest while the mother bird is on it, and commands that we remove the mother bird first.[4] Maimonides, in his *Guide for the Perplexed*' explains some of these laws as follows: "It is likewise forbidden to slaughter an animal and its young on the same day. This is a precautionary measure to avoid slaughtering the young animal in front of its mother. For in the cases animals feel very great pain, there being no difference regarding this pain between man and the other animals. But the love and the tenderness of a mother for her child is not consequent upon reason, but upon the activity of the imaginative faculty, which is found in most animals just as it is found in man. This law applies in particular to ox and lamb, because these are the domestic animals that we are allowed to eat and that in most cases it is usual to eat . . . . This is also the reason for the commandment to chase the mother bird away from the nest before taking the fledglings."[5]

The Midrashic commentaries on the Bible contain many Rabbinic statements which indicate that kindness to animals is an absolute requirement. Moses and David were chosen as leaders because God noted their gentle and understanding treatment of their flocks.[6]

Despite these prohibitions against cruelty towards animals, Judaism does not agree with anti-vivisection statutes which bar animal experimentation. Animals were created for the benefit of human beings and may be used for food and as beasts of burden. Vegetarianism is thus not generally regarded as a form of exemplary piety. Animals may be used for other purposes as well, even though utilization for such purposes results in incidental pain to the animal, e.g., feathers may be removed for use as quills. Unnecessary pain, however, is forbidden.

---

4. Deut. 25:4, Lev. 22:28, Gen. 9:4, and Deut. 12:23, 22:10, 22:6–7.
5. Maimonides, Guide for the Perplexed, 3:48.
6. Midrash Rabbah Exodus, 2:2.

The fundamental criterion establishing a line of demarkation between the permissable and the forbidden is the relationship of the act involved to a legitimate human need. Cruelty for its own sake or for the sake of sport is always forbidden. Rabbinic authorities have interpreted that hunting as a sport is forbidden for precisely that reason. Scientific experiments upon laboratory animals designed to yield information of potential benefit to mankind are permitted in Jewish Law as legitimate utilization of animals for the tangible b efit of mankind. Of course pain may be inflicted upon the animal only to the degree absolutely necessary in order to obtain the required information. Otherwise the pain does not serve to satisfy a legitimate need and is prohibited.

It should be stressed that this criterion is a pragmatic one. The benefits must be practical in nature and not simply the satisfaction of intellectual curiosity. Thus, while animal research by scientists is justified, and while surgical skills may be perfected through practice on animals, a teacher should not demand that a student perform experiments which inflict pain upon animals unless the experiment is directly related to the development of a specific skill necessary for fulfilment of the student's professional vocational goal of alleviating human pain or suffering.

On the basis of this discussion it can be clearly seen that use of animals for food or for clothing is not prohibited by Jewish Law, just as the use of animals for experimentation that would lead to the benefit of mankind is not forbidden. Wanton killing, such as in hunting animals not harmful to man for sport, is wrong. In all cases, inflicting unnecessary pain on an animal is contrary to Jewish Law. In fact, while the procedure of kosher slaughter is specifically mandated in the Bible, studies of the method show it to be the most humane method in existence for slaughtering an animal. Thus, with the swift stroke of a razor sharp, therefore painless knife, the carotid arteries as well as esophagus and trachea are severed instantly, thus causing the animal immediate and painless loss of consciousness.

In summary, the Chief Rabbi, adhering to the laws and guidelines of Judaism, cannot outlaw the use of animals for human need and consumption. For Judaism regards the animal kingdom as having been created to serve humankind. But Judaism does prohibit inflicting unnecessary, cruel or wanton pain on animals, not only in trapping them, but in all man's relationship of responsibility for them such as with pets and domestic animals. It opposed hunting for sport as well, because that, too, inflicts unnecessary pain and is considered cruel.

7

The York Question

Q**uestion** (From the Managing Editor, York Archaeological Trust for Excavation and Research, Picadilly House, York): As you know, March 16/17, 1190, were the dates of the mass suicide of the Jews of ancient York, who chose death rather than fall into the hands of the mob besieging the castle in which they had taken refuge against the threat of conversion or death. A few Jews remained in York till the final expulsion of all Jews from England in 1290. After Jews returned to England in the latter part of the seventeenth century, religious Jews continued to shun York because they did not know exactly where the remains of those martyrs lay in the city. Recent archeological discoveries have pinpointed the Jewish cemetery and other remains, and in conformity with the requirements of Judaism, all remains which had not been properly buried were suitably interred, despite the desire of medical researchers and biological scientists to be permitted to use parts of the remains for research. Because of this conformance with the requirements of Judaism, religious Jews have now resumed visiting the city.[1]

It has come to my attention that certain microscopic particles of plaque from the teeth of some of the victims were taken by a researcher and not yet buried. Must they be buried as the bones had been? If not, may these microscopic pieces or traces of plaque be used for research and study?

Answer: There are two issues which must be considered. The first is the proper burial of Jewish remains, and particles of bone are considered remains and must be buried. Thus, if there are any particles of tooth material included or embedded in the plaque, they must be buried. That is, however, according to your description, quite unlikely. Bone must be buried, and plaque is not bone though tooth particles are. Microscopic pieces or traces would, under ordinary circumstances, not be of concern to us. A particle of tooth material which can be seen and handled, is.

There is another consideration. According to Jewish law, it is forbidden to have any benefit from a corpse. This is obviously an issue here. In the spirit of this concern is an additional question. Can we derive benefit from data derived from martyrs?

This is an issue which scientists have debated in connection with the data amassed by the Nazis on the basis of their infamous human experiments. While there are some who seek

---

1. I had checked into the question of visiting York. There was no specific prohibition or herem enacted by the rabbis to prevent such visitation. There was a custom which had arisen based on the rabbinic prohibition to walk in an area which possibly contained an unmarked grave or body part (Mishnah, Ohalot 2:1, Maimonides, Mishneh Torah, 2:16). Since the graves of many of the martyrs were unknown, Jews were reluctant to visit York. When the graves of the martyrs had recently become known, pious Jews no longer had any reason to avoid York.

to permit use of such data, many scientists and ethicists find its use abhorrent.[2] Jewish authorities have tended to prohibit the publication and use of such data.

It goes without saying that the action of the scientist-researcher who gathered the plaque cannot be equated with the Nazis and their villainy. But we must accept the fact that he gathered the information without authorization, and such an action would be in the category of deriving benefit from corpses. It might be argued that the particles are microscopic and normally Judaism overlooks prohibited matter which is not visible to the naked eye. Technically, this is true. The martyrs of York, however, can be considered an exception, since their martyrdom was an act of religious persecution and anti-Semitism. In such cases the particles should not be used, just as in the case of the Nazi experiments, even pure data without remnants of the original martyrs, should not be used.

---

2. Arthur Caplan, Monstrous Medicine, papers presented at a 1988 conference on "The Meaning of the Holocaust for Bioethics."

Index

About the Author

Nisson E. Shulman has served as a rabbi in leading congregations on three continents: New York's Fifth Avenue Synagogue, Sydney, Australia's Central Synagogue, and London's St. John Wood Synagogue, the flagship congregation of the United Synagogue (Orthodox) of Great Britain. He is the author of *Authority and Community*, which recreates the community of Central Europe from where most Ashkenazic Jews are descended. A former editor of the *Medical Ethics Yearbook for London's Jew's College*, Rabbi Shulman currently serves as the Director of the Department of Rabbinic Services of the Max Stern Department of Communal Services, RIETS, Yeshiva University in New York City. He served on the Commission on Medical Ethics of the Federation of Jewish Philanthropies, New York City, and resides in Manhattan with his wife, Rywka.